ORGAN DONATION: SUPPLY, POLICIES AND PRACTICES

ORGAN DONATION: SUPPLY, POLICIES AND PRACTICES

PETR T. GRINKOVSKIY
EDITOR

Nova Science Publishers, Inc.
New York

For permission to use material from this book please contact us:
Telephone 631-231-7269; Fax 631-231-8175
Web Site: http://www.novapublishers.com

LIBRARY OF CONGRESS CATALOGING-IN-PUBLICATION DATA
Available upon request
ISBN: 978-1-60692-501-0

Published by Nova Science Publishers, Inc. ✢ New York

CONTENTS

PREFACE

The issue of living organ donation is important because it represents one important set of possibilities for balancing the needs of people seeking organs with one another, and with the needs of potential organ donors. On one side of the balance, the drive to increase the supply of transplantable organs is fueled by people awaiting organ transplants. They are, in a sense, competing with one another on waiting lists for potentially life-saving scarce resources. On the other side of the balance, the drive to ensure that the transplant system is ethical and equitable precludes some mechanisms that would increase the supply of transplantable organs. Some options that have been rejected to date in the United States include paying healthy persons to donate their organs, and mandating that transplantable organs be harvested from all cadavers. To maintain the most ideal balance for the organ transplantation system, Congress may now wish to clarify whether certain new types of living organ donation should be adopted to increase the supply of transplantable organs, or prohibited for ethical and/or equitable reasons.

In: Organ Donation: Supply, Policies and Practices ISBN: 978-1-60692-501-0
Editor: P. T. Grinkovskiy

Chapter 1

ORGAN DONATION: UTILIZING PUBLIC POLICY AND TECHNOLOGY TO STRENGTHEN ORGAN DONOR PROGRAMS*

Statement of

James Burdick
Division of Transplantation Healthcare Systems Bureau

Good afternoon Mr. Chairman, Members of the Subcommittee. Thank you for the opportunity to meet with you today on behalf of the Health Resources and Services Administration (HRSA) to discuss the roles and responsibilities of the Division of Transplantation in strengthening our nation's organ donor programs and awareness activities. I appreciate your continuing support of the organ donation and transplantation programs.

---

* This is an edited, excerpted and augmented publication of a U.S. Department of Health and Human Services Statement dated September 25, 2007.

BACKGROUND

The need for organ transplants continues to grow and this demand continues to outpace the supply of transplantable organs. Nineteen people in this country will die every day because a life-saving organ does not become available to them.

During the past decade, the number of deceased donors increased between 2-3 percent annually while the annual growth rate in the number of individuals waiting for an organ transplant increased by approximately 8 percent. Even with the recent unprecedented 10.8 percent increase in the number of deceased donors in 2004, followed by a 6.2 percent increase in 2005, there were still about 97,000 individuals waiting for an organ transplant at the end of 2006.

HRSA is responsible for administering a number of organ donation and transplantation programs. The National Organ Transplant Act (NOTA) (P.L. 98-507), as amended, authorized the creation and operation of: (1) the Organ Procurement and Transplantation Network (OPTN), operated under contract with HRSA, which facilitates the matching of donor organs with individuals waiting for an organ transplant; (2) the operation of the Scientific Registry of Transplant Recipients (SRTR), which facilitates the ongoing evaluation of the scientific and clinical status of organ transplantation; and (3) grants and contracts to conduct projects designed to increase the number of organ donors.

Additional program authorities were provided by the Organ Donation and Recovery Improvement Act (ODRIA) (P.L. 108-2 16), which amended NOTA, to help increase the number of organ donors and number of organs made available for transplantation. The key additional authorities under ODRIA include: (1) grants to States to support organ donation awareness programs; (2) grants and contracts to support public education and outreach activities designed to increase the number of organ donors, including living donors; (3) grants to qualified organ procurement organizations and hospitals to establish programs to increase the rate of organ donation; (4) the expansion of grant making authority to include public institutions; (5) the development and dissemination of educational materials to inform health care professionals and other appropriate professionals about organ, tissue and eye donation; (6) financial assistance to living donors to help defray travel and other incidental non-medical expenses; and (7) mechanisms to evaluate the long-term effects of living organ donation.

CURRENT ACTIVITIES

In 2006, a total of 28,923 organ transplant operations were performed nationwide, up from 28,112 the year before. From the 2006 operations, 31,184 organs were transplanted; of that number, 24,461 organs came from deceased donors (78.4 percent), and 6,723 transplanted organs were from living donors (21.6 percent).

At HRSA, one of the ways we are keeping donation efforts on a fast track is through our highly successful Organ Donation Breakthrough Collaborative. The Collaborative brings together donation professionals and hospital leaders to identify and share best practices to maximize organ donation rates in their facilities. Some of the Collaborative outcomes include: Hospital-Organ Procurement Organization (OPO) teambuilding, increased donors after cardiac death, and increased conversion rates and donors in non-Collaborative hospitals. The goal is to raise donation rates to 75 percent of eligible organ donors. The results are most impressive: since 2003, the number of hospitals that have achieved the 75 percent goal has increased from 55 to 301.

To complement the Organ Donation Breakthrough Collaborative, the Organ Transplantation Breakthrough Collaborative was initiated in October 2005. This Collaborative is designed to make more organs available for transplantation by increasing the average number of organs retrieved from each donor. The goal of this Collaborative is to increase the number of organs transplanted from deceased donors by 22.6 percent.

This year, HHS joined with private companies and organizations across America in encouraging their employees to "Give Five-Save Lives." The "Give Five-Save Lives" challenge asked employees to support donation by taking five minutes out of their workday to enroll in a State organ donor registry or sign a donor card.

"Give Five-Save Lives" grew out of our Workplace Partnership for Life program, which today includes more than 11,000 workplace partners committed to addressing the shortage of transplantable organs. Through this Workplace Initiative, more than 400,000 individuals signified their intent to be organ donors in State registries over the 2006 holiday season from Thanksgiving to the New Year.

In February, HRSA announced the results of a 2005 Gallup Organization survey which indicates that Americans continue to strongly support the donation of organs and tissues for transplantation. More important, the survey also found that 52.3 percent of Americans have taken personal actions to become organ donors since a similar 1993 survey on donation.

Donor families want things to proceed the best way possible to have some good come out of tragedy. Consistent with our efforts to increase organ donation, there are strong safeguards in place to ensure that life-saving care of the critically ill patient comes first. There is a strict prohibition against the transplant team participating in the care of the patient who is a potential donor. There is also a thorough consent process which includes time for the family to think about and discuss the decision, and donation can only proceed with a signed consent. Three IOM reports have supported the value of donation after cardiac death, when appropriate.

Last month, HRSA announced grant winners under the State Donor Registry Support Program. The grants help States without a registry to develop one, and help those States with a registry to make enhancements to keep pace with technology and new information. The aim of the program is to help ensure that all U.S. residents have an opportunity to indicate and store their donation wishes where they can be reliably retrieved at their time of death.

HRSA currently operates two demonstration grant programs designed to increase knowledge about practices that are effective in increasing the number of organs available for transplantation. The Social and Behavioral Interventions to Increase Organ and Tissue Donation grant program funds projects to implement and evaluate social and behavioral studies to increase family consent to donation and/or individual intent to donate. The Clinical Interventions to Increase Organ Procurement grant program focuses on clinical activities that begin after consent is determined or given at time of death and extend until transplantation. Improving these clinical activities influence whether a particular donor actually progresses to become a donor and the number and quality of organs that may be procured for transplantation.

HRSA also awarded a cooperative agreement to the Regents of the University of Michigan with a subcontract to the American Society of Transplant Surgeons to provide support for reimbursement of travel and subsistence expenses incurred toward living organ donation with priority given to those potential donors without the financial means to pay these expenses.

Three hundred twenty-three hospitals have recently won the Department's Medal of Honor for substantially raising the organ donation rates of eligible donors from their facilities. The ceremony to congratulate these hospitals will be held this October in Tennessee.

Despite these advances, HRSA is humbled by the fact that people are still dying because of the lack of available organs. In our vigilance, HRSA sustains support for other organ donation programs. The OPTN, which HRSA manages, continues to improve the efficiency of the organ transplantation system by improving organ allocation policies and monitoring policy compliance by transplant programs and OPOs. Grants were awarded to OPOs and hospitals to establish program coordinating organ donation activities. In our outreach efforts, HRSA maintains support for public and professional education programs.

HRSA is pleased that, in response to a Departmental request, the Department of Justice's Office of the Legal Counsel (OLC) issued an opinion on March 28, 2007 concerning the proper interpretation of the criminal prohibition on organ transfers for "valuable consideration" in section 301 of NOTA. The OLC concluded that paired exchanges and living donor/deceased donor exchanges do not involve "valuable consideration" under section 301 and are therefore not prohibited under this statute. The published opinion is binding on U.S. Attorneys' offices (which have the primary role in enforcing Federal criminal laws, such as section 301). Because of this opinion, concerns about the legality of paired exchanges or of living donor/deceased donor exchanges have been resolved, enabling the OPTN contractor to operate a nationwide paired exchange system. We believe that this will result in hundreds of additional lives saved each year.

Working together, we are making great strides, but we still have a long way to go.

Future Activities

HRSA is always looking for new and better ways to increase the number of organ donors and donor awareness. Some major activities underway include:

Breakthrough Collaboratives

Both the Organ Donation Breakthrough Collaborative and the Organ Transplantation Breakthrough Collaborative are designed to rapidly spread best practices of organ procurement organizations and donor hospitals to increase the number of deceased donors and to increase the number of organs made available for transplantation from each deceased donor. We will continue these efforts.

Our most recent initiative is the Transplant Growth and Management Collaborative. The goal of this collaborative is to save or enhance thousands of lives a year by maximizing the number of organs transplanted from each and every donor and building the necessary capacity within the Nation's transplant programs to transplant 35,000 organs annually. Elements of the Initiative include: a best practices study (December 2006 – February 2007), expert panel meeting (May 2007) and a Transplant Center Growth and Management Collaborative (to be launched in October 2007). *Organ Procurement and Transplantation Network (OPTN)*

The OPTN is working to revise the national kidney/kidney-pancreas allocation policy to optimize net lifetime survival benefit of kidney/kidney-pancreas transplantation. Additionally, the OPTN is working to improve the information technology and operations infrastructure of the OPTN to allow more rapid and efficient placement of deceased donor organs.

Scientific Registry of Transplant Recipients (SRTR)

The SRTR conducts analyses of information for all organ donors and transplant recipients to be used for public and professional information and policy making purposes.

Organ Donation Support

The program will continue to test new approaches to increase the number of donors as well as the number and quality of donor organs for transplantation. We are looking for approaches that yield results.

Public and Professional Education Programs

The programs will continue to promote organ and tissue donation through a variety of initiatives targeted to the general public and to medical and other professionals who are influential in the organ donation process. We must continue to get the word out.

CONCLUSION

While nearly 29,000 individuals received life-saving transplants in 2006, the need to increase the number of successful transplants remains critical. There are close to 97,000 patients on the national waiting list to receive an organ, and 19 will die every day because a life-saving organ does not become available to them.

Working together, we can change these numbers. HRSA is proud of its leadership role in this most worthwhile effort. There are clear signs we are moving in the right direction, but we must do everything we can to keep the momentum going.

Thank you for giving me the opportunity to come here today to discuss the organ donation and transplantation, and for your dedication and interest in these vital programs. I would be happy to answer any questions you have.

In: Organ Donation: Supply, Policies and Practices ISBN: 978-1-60692-501-0
Editor: P. T. Grinkovskiy © 2009 Nova Science Publishers, Inc.

Chapter 2

INFORMATION POLICY, CENSUS, AND NATIONAL ARCHIVES SUBCOMMITTEE, OVERSIGHT AND GOVERNMENT REFORM COMMITTEE, "ORGAN DONATION: UTILIZING PUBLIC POLICY AND TECHNOLOGY TO STRENGHTHEN ORGAN DONOR PROGRAMS"*

Testimony of

Clive 0. Callender

Minority Organ Tissue Transplant Education Program

The number one problem in transplantation today is the shortage of donors. More than 96,000 people today are on transplant waiting lists. Nearly 25,000 transplants are performed annually leaving an organ donor recipient disparity of 65,000. This disparity results in nearly 20 deaths/day at least seven of which are African Americans (A.A.). In order to answer the questions, what has happened to organ donations in the A.A. population, and how it compares with donations in other ethnic groups? I will share three decades of work (1982-

* This is an edited, excerpted and augmented Information Policy, Census, and National Archives Subcommittee Testimony dated September 25, 2007.

2005) in the African American community which have culminated in the development of a methodology which has narrowed the A.A. donor gap, and which has the potential to help narrow or eliminate other minority health disparities. African Americans represent 13% of the American population, but make up 35% of those on kidney transplant waiting lists. In 1982 when we began our first African American donation campaign, it was stated that Blacks "don't and won't" donate organs for transplant purposes. Then the A.A. donations rate in organ donors per million (O.D.M.) was eight compared to eighteen O.D.M. in the Caucasian population. We then began the D.C. Organ Donor Program (DCODP) in conjunction with Howard University and the National Kidney Foundation of the National Capital Area between 1982 and 1990 with five hundred dollars from Howard University. This program began with a two hour community focus group session with forty District of Columbia residents and included one kidney donor and one transplant recipient. Upon completion of these sessions, we identified the five commonest obstacles to organ donation in the District of Columbia. They were: 1). Lack of transplant awareness, 2). Religious myths and misperceptions, 3). Medical distrust, 4). Fear of premature death after signing a donor card, 5). Racism. The second important outcome of those focus sessions was that while only two of forty had signed donor cards at the beginning of the session, forty of forty donor cards were signed by the end of the session. This led us to form the DCODP in August of 1982; this was a grass roots effort to change behavior in the District and the surrounding Metropolitan Washington area. The cultural and ethnically sensitive presentations to the community were directed at overcoming the five obstacles identified above

By 1990 the number of donor cards signed at the D.C. Motor Vehicle Office increased from 25/month to 750/month and the number of A.A. organ donors in the District of Columbia doubled. Because of the success of the DCODP, the Dow Chemical Company (1986-1992) sponsored my involvement in national media tours in fifty cities to increase awareness about the need for more Black donors. This initiative merged the community grass roots, face-to-face interaction and mass media approach. Gallup Polls done in 1985 and 1990 identified that the number of Blacks aware of the highly successful nature of transplants and the number of Blacks signing donor cards had tippled during this five year period secondary to this Dow Chemical Company Take Initiative Program directed at the A.A. population. This led us to conceptualize The National Minority Organ Tissue Transplant Education Program (MOTTEP) in 1991 to use this successful community grass root and mass media approach in all minority groups (African American, Latino/Hispanic, Asian, Pacific Islander, Alaskan Native, American Indian).

Congressman Louis Stokes, Secretary of Health and Human Services, Dr. Louis Sullivan and Dr. John Ruffin then intervened and encouraged us to seek NTH funding to allow for the development of fifteen community grass root programs in fifteen cities across the United States (Anchorage, Alaska; Birmingham, Alabama; Los Angeles, California; Washington, D.C.; Miami, Florida; Atlanta, Georgia; Honolulu, Hawaii; Chicago, Illinois; Detroit, Michigan; Albuquerque, New Mexico; Brooklyn, New York; Cleveland, Ohio; Nashville, Tennessee; Houston, Texas; and Richmond, Virginia).

What Is the National MOTTEP Model?

The National MOTTEP model was conceptualized based upon the successes of our previous African American education programs such as the local DC Organ Donor Project (DCODP), 1982-1988 and nationally, the DOW Chemical Company Take Initiative Program (DOWTIP), 1986-1992. These successes led us to utilize their successful methodologies with the Latino- Hispanic, Native American, Alaskan Native and Asian-Pacific Islander populations as the National Minority Organ Tissue Transplant Education Program (MOTTEP). This model combines media campaigns and grass roots efforts to disseminate a two-pronged message: preventing chronic diseases particularly hypertension, renal failure, diabetes and obesity while simultaneously increasing organ donation rates. The following is a summarization of the national impact of MOTTEP.

A 25 Year Data Analysis of a National Donor Education Program

Since 1982 we have participated in a national donor education program emphasizing community education and empowerment requiring the community to be an efficient change agent. As described above, the grass roots approach is combined with mass media aimed to: 1) increase organ donation rates and 2) adopt healthy lifestyle behaviors. The methodology utilizes culturally sensitive and ethnically similar community individuals who are transplant recipients, donors and their family members as messengers. Three distinct eras are evident.

Era I — 1982 —	Present Era II — 1995-2005	Era III — 1995-2005
'African American Impact	Hispanic/Latino Impact	Asian Impact

A review of National African American data demonstrated a change from 8 organ donors/million (1982) to 40.8 organ donors/million (2002). A 50 city campaign Gallup Poll (1986-1992) demonstrated a tripling of Black awareness of the success of transplants and the number of Blacks signing donor cards. Locally, donor card signings increased from 25/month to 750/month (1982-1988) and Black donors in the District of Columbia doubled by 1988. Tables 1-3 illustrate increases in donors, donation rates, organ donors/million and the impact on donation rates in cities with a national structured effort versus areas those cities without a national effort.

Table 1. Minorities Donate in Proportion to their Population Distribution

Ethnicity	(Population Percentage (2003)	[Donation Percentage
Black	112.7	12.6
Hispanic	110.9	12.2
Asian	0.8 1	2

CADAVERIC DONORS PER 1,000 EVALUABLE DEATHS AND NUMBER OF DONORS BY ETHNICITY AND OPO'S, 1995-1998

Table 2.

	MOTTEP		Non MOTTEP		
Ethnicity	Donation Rate	Donors	Donation Rate	Donors	p-value
White, Non Hispanic	59.3	A ,928	59.2	11,279	0.02
White, Hispanic	106.9	1,055	47.4	886	<.01
Black	43.4	1,263	32.9	1,286	<.01
Other	50.7	228	A2.4	272	<.01

Table 3.

	Number of Donors		Donors/Million		Donation Percentages	
Ethnicity	1999	2000	1990	2000	2000	2005
Black	659	1373	22,4	40,8	11.2%	14%
Hispanic/Latino	518	1319	22,9	40,2	11,2%	13,2%
Asian	73	278	10,3	26,2	2,7%	2,6%
Minority Donor Total					25,1%	30% (29,8%)

NATIONAL MOTTEP'S PAST ACCOMPLISHMENTS

In the past, National MOTTEP® has used several intervention mechanisms that, because of their success, will be used in our expanded programs. First, MOTTEP® has made extensive use of the media in order to change minority behavior regarding organ and tissue donation and about healthy living. For example, media impressions between 1993 and 2006 have increased from 30 million to more than 8 billion respectively. By reaching an average of one million community persons annually, National MOTTEP has empowered communities to meet the challenge head on by participating in the donor process and adopting healthy lifestyles to prevent the need for transplantation. The figure below lists some milestones throughout MOTTEP's history. Through the expanded efforts, MOTTEP anticipates creating new milestones.

MOTTEP MILESTONES

I.A. 1991 — 1993

- MOTTEP Conceptualized in 1991 — Callender/Smith.
- MOTTEP Concept and Strategic Plan — Sponsored by Congressman Louis Stokes — 1992.
- MOTTEP authorization approved by Congressional Appropriations Committee — May 1992. MOTTEP legislation authorized by President Bush in the Fall of 1992.
- Development of an African American Strategic Plan.
- Development of a Hispanic Strategic Plan.

I.B. 1993 —1995

- First MOTTEP contract from office of the NIH Director, Dr. Bernadine Healy, and Dr. John
- Ruffin, Associate Director, NIH Office of Minority Health Research — 1993 to 1995.
- Development of MOTTEP survey evaluation tool — Pre & Post MOTTEP presentations.
- Organ Donation: The Problem; MOTTEP: The Solution — This publication chronicles MOTTEP' s evolution.
- Development of National African American Transplant Strategic Plan.
- Development of National Latino Transplant Strategic Plan.
- Development of MOTTEP "Give to Save" Logo and Theme Song.
- Appeared on the Oprah Winfrey Show, BET, CBS Evening News — all national TV shows with audiences exceeding 9 million.
- "Focus on Health" weekly radio talk show on WOL (Washington, DC and Baltimore, MD) from 1993 to 1995.

II. 1995 to 1999

- National Minority Transplant Hall of Fame Inaugurated — September 1, 1996.
- Inaugurated National Minority Donor Awareness Day — August 1, 1996.
- Evaluation reports on findings of the program effectiveness study using data from matched sets of pre- and post- questionnaires for all youth and adult participants showed that: 1) statistically significant increases ($P<0.5$) occurred in the levels of knowledge on organ/tissue donation; and 2) participants significantly more likely to state their willingness to become organ/tissue donors after hearing the MOTTEP presentations.
- Implementation of the First National Model Minority Transplant Strategic Plan — 1995.
- Implementation of the First National Latino Transplant Strategic Plan — 1995.
- Developed the First National Asian-Pacific Islander Transplant Strategic Plan — 1995.
- Developed the First National Minority Community Transplant Information Resource Center — 1995.

- Under the influence of MOTTEP, African American organ donors per million (O.D.M.) increased from 8 in 1982 to 20 O.D.M. in 1995 and to 28 O.D.M. in 1998.
- Likewise, Hispanic/Latino O.D.M. increased from 9 in 1994 to 18 in 1998.
- During this same time period, Asian/Pacific Islander O.D.M. doubled.
- African American/Black recipients of African American/Black organ donors increased from 3% in 1985 to 23% in 1998.
- Total Number of Media Impressions from July 1, 1995 — 1999; 3 Billion.
- Total Number of People Reached Through Face-to-Face Presentations since July 1, 1995 equaled 4 Million.
- Generated 492 publications and presentations; 46 academic publications and 23 videos;
- Total number of requests for materials — 1009.
- Organ and Tissue Donations Directly Linked To MOTTEP Presentations As of June 1, 1999:
- 38 donors from MOTTEP presentations. Birmingham — 2 donations (4/2/98 and 1/3/99); Atlanta — 2 donations, Detroit — 2 donations (1/29/99 and 5/28/99), Honolulu — 1 donation (1/99), Nashville — 1 donation (5/12/99), Chicago/NW Indiana — 30 donations (since beginning of grant in 1995).
- Total number of pre/post surveys (youth and adult) — 7048.
- The number of National or International — publications on MOTTEP and minority transplant education efforts since 1995 is thirty.
- Two Institute of Medicine presentations 1999; one presentation to Secretary Shalala's "Forum on Liver Allocation and Organ Donation" — 1996; two MOTTEP presentations (testimonies) before the Congress of the United States (April 18 and June 18, 1999).
- Development Of The First National Minority Donation Education effort — Community-based with a grass roots and multimedia combined approach — 1993.
- Produced and Hosted "Focus on Health" — a weekly two-hour radio call-in talk show on WOL (Washington, DC and Baltimore, MD) ---1993 to 1995.
- MOTTEP modus operandus identifies — donors and donor families, transplant recipients, transplant candidates of local community origin and ethnically and culturally similar and sensitive — as the most effective messengers — 1993 to 1995.

Other "Firsts" Accomplishments Include (1993-1995):

- First to identify community as the most potent and cost efficient "change agent" — 1993 to
- 1995.
- First to emphasize the importance of the combination of "Prevent the Need" and "Increased
- Need for Organ/Tissue Donors" as the most efficient mode of community outreach and education (1993-1995).
- Implementation of the First Model National Minority Transplant Strategic Plan.
- Implementation of the First National Latino/Hispanic Transplant Strategic Plan.
- Developed the First National Asian and Pacific Islander Transplant Strategic Plan.
- First to identify community as the most potent and cost efficient "change agent".
- First to emphasize the importance of simultaneously promoting the messages of "Preventing
- the Need" and "Increasing the Number of Organ/Tissue Donors" as the most efficient mode of community transplant-related outreach.
- First to take the fruits of the first minority donor education programs of the District of Columbia Organ Donor Program (DCODP) and the Dow Chemical Company Take Initiative Program (DOWTIP), and apply them to all ethnic minority groups via funding by the National Institutes of Health — Office of Research on Minority Health and the National Institutes on Diabetes and Digestive and Kidney Diseases (1993).
- First to inaugurate National Minority Donor Awareness Day (August 1, 1996).
- First to establish the National Minority Transplant Hall of Fame (September 1, 1996).

As previously mentioned, National MOTTEP was the first program of its kind in the country that was designed to: I) educate minority communities on facts about organ/tissue transplants and how to maintain the health of key organs and tissues; 2) empower minority communities to develop programs to increase awareness; and 3) increase minority participation in organ/tissue transplant endeavors including signing organ donor cards, encouraging family discussions and involving parents in the decision to retain the health of kidneys, livers, hearts, lungs and other organs.

National MOTTEP was also one of the first organizations in the country to work to expand its original grassroots efforts to include a health promotion and disease prevention component that exclusively targeted youth as well as adults. The disease prevention aspect was added to decrease the disproportionate rate of hypertension, diabetes and other diseases that affect minority populations. More specifically, a comprehensive, intensive outreach campaign focused upon uncontrolled or untreated diabetes mellitus, hypertension, proper nutrition, increased physical activity and avoiding the use of alcohol and other substances by minorities.

However, National MOTTEP's primary activities have remained the design, implementation, and evaluation of educational programs for national use in order to increase the number of minority Americans who take active roles in organ and tissue donation and who hold family discussions. National MOTTEP also provided leadership in educating the public about how to maintain sound organs. To support these campaigns, MOTTEP utilized the following strategies: Established networks of speakers, (i.e., youth, parents, celebrities, transplant recipients, donor family members, transplant candidates, health care professionals) who were available to religious and community-based organizations to promote organ and tissue health; Identified, accessed and utilized print media and radio technology to increase awareness among minority audiences of organ and tissue health; Supported and sponsored national and local forums which targeted public, private and community leaders who then disseminated information to minority communities on organ and tissue health; Established a library of audiotapes, videotapes, print and other materials which were made available for duplication; Followed up on any media coverage related to organ and tissue health to generate a greater knowledge of issues related to organ/tissue health; and Collaborated with an exceptionally large range of other community-based organizations in order to implement health promotion and public awareness campaigns at each of the sites in the targeted cities.

MOTTEP of HONOLULU - Accomplishments

The goal of this project is to expand educational efforts across all ethnic, religious and age groups to increase the number of individuals consenting to donate organs and tissues and to increase the supply of organs for waiting transplant recipients through the expansion of a public education program on organ and tissue donation.

The Minority Organ Tissue Transplant Education Program (MOTTEP) is a nationwide program designed to educate ethnic minority communities about organ and tissue donation and transplantation to increase the number of donations from these communities. The Organ Donor Center of Hawaii (ODCH) implemented MOTTEP of Hawaii in 1995. The program currently focuses on Hawaii's local Filipino community which had the highest number of individuals on the organ transplant waiting list {36%) and the lowest number consenting to donation {3%). In 2002, the University of Hawaii — Cancer Research Center of Hawaii (CRCH), in collaboration with ODCH and various Filipino community organization was awarded a five-year grant to continue MOTTEP. Funding of the program will end in June, 2007.

The program's objectives, as it remains focused on the Filipino community and extends its outreach to Hawaiian and Pacific Islander communities, are to:

- Increase the number of individuals designating themselves as organ donors via driver's license, state ID and/or donor card
- Assure that family discussions occur to inform their loved ones of their wishes
- Increase the number family consents for organ and tissue donation
- Increase education and awareness about organ and tissue donation in the community.

Organ Donor Center of Hawaii will continue to focus on Filipino community and plans to expand the MOTTEP to the Hawaiian and Pacific Islander Communities. Currently 49 of the 375 Hawaii residents on the Hawaii Transplant Waitlist are Pacific Islanders, the second largest group after Asians (which include Filipinos) who represent the largest ethnic group in the waitlist. Over the past 3 years, the Hawaiian and Pacific Islander groups represent the third largest potential organ donor group, but the lowest consenting ethnic group.

Since implementation in 1995, the Organ Donor Center of Hawaii has been working within the Filipino community through MOTTEP. The program's success is documented through an increase in the Filipino donor consent from 3% to 27% during that time period. Over the past 3 years, organ donation consent rates among Filipinos have steadily increased: 40% in 2004, 67% in 2005, and 71% in 2006. It is evident that MOTTEP's public education efforts to improve organ donation rates among the Filipino population have been effective and we wish to sustain this success. The result of this successful program is evidenced in increased donor consent in the Filipino community from 3% to 71%.

MOTTEP is a national model that has shown to be culturally effective in the Filipino Community and will be adapted and expanded to include other Hawaiian Pacific Islander communities.

SUMMARY

Since 1982 we have participated in the growth and development of a national donor education program which relies on a grass roots strategy that emphasizes community education and empowerment requiring the community to be an efficient and economically appropriate change agent.

Methodolgy

The data presented provide compelling evidence of the efficiency of a community-based grass roots approach combined with mass media to deliver a two-pronged message aimed at: 1) increasing organ donation rates and 2) promoting the adoption of healthy lifestyle behaviors and practices. The key for its success is utilizing a methodology emphasizing the use of culturally sensitive and ethnically similar community individuals who are transplant recipients, donors and their family members as messengers. Three distinct eras are evident.

Era I —1982 — Present	Era II — 1995-2005	Era HI — 1995-2005
African American Impact	Hispanic/Latino Impact	Asian Impact

Results

African American data emphasized here reflects the impact of national education efforts resulting in an increase from 8 organ donors/million (1982) to 40.8 organ donors/million (2002). Regionally, a 50 city campaign Gallup Poll (1986-1992) demonstrates a tripling of Black awareness of the success of transplants and the number of Blacks signing donor cards. Locally, the number of donor cards signed increased from 25/month to 750/month (1982-1988) and the number of Black donors in the District of Columbia doubled by 1988. Tables 1-3 below illustrate the increases in donors, donation rates, organ donors/million and the impact on donation rates with a national structured effort versus areas without a national effort.

Table 1. Minorities Donate in Proportion to their Population Distribution

Ethnicity	Population Rate	Donation Rate
White	71.7	72.1
Black	12.7	12.6
Hispanic	10.9	12.2
Asian	3.8	2

CADAVERIC DONORS PER 1,000 EVALUABLE DEATHS AND NUMBER OF DONORS BY ETHNICITY AND OPO'S, 1995-1998

Table 2.

	National Effort		No National Effort		value
Ethnicity	Donation Rate	Donors	Donation Rate	Donors	
White, Non Hispanic	59.3	4,928	59.2	11,279	0.02
White, Hispanic	105.9	1,055	47.4	886	<.01
Black	43.4	1,263	32.9	1,286	<.01
Other	50.7	228	42.4	272	<.01

Table 3.

	Number of Donors		Organ Donors/Million		Donation %	
Ethnicity	1990	2000	1990	2000	2000	2005
Black	659	1373	22.4	40.8	11.2%	14%
Hispanic/Latino	518	1319	22.9	40.2	11.2%	13.2%
Asian	73	278	10.3	26.2	2.7%	2.6%

CONCLUSION

Since the half lives for kidney transplants range from 5.3 (A.A.) to 12.2 (Asian), and 50% of all grafts survive at least 5 years and most more than 9 years, it is clear that the financial benefit to the government supporting a national donor education program such as this would save millions of dollars. Since outpatient dialysis costs are in excess of $40,000.00/yr per patient and transplants break even after 3 years, this would provide an average savings of at least $30,000.00/yr for each year the grafts survives over 3 years. Assuming a graft survival rate of 6 years, each donor (living or deceased) organ would save at least $135,000.00 per donor (1.5 x $30,000.00 x 3 years. Deceased donors provide an average of 3 organs/donor while living donors provide 1 organ/donor). Assuming out patient kidney transplant costs after 3 years = $10,000.00/yr, looking at the graphics presented above, it is clear that the cost benefit ratio of a model national donor education program such as the one presented here is a worthy investment whose benefits greatly outweigh the under-funded support currently provided.

These data are based upon the current census that identifies 25% of the American population as minorities. The MOTTEP goal is by 2010 to have 35% of the donors being minorities and to have African Americans (A.A.) and Latino O.D.M. to increase from 41 O.D. M. to 50 O.D.M. This would allow for the recovery of 1750 minority donor organs and save the Government 236 million dollars.

While MOTTEP has received a total of $16 million dollars from the Federal Government between 1992 and now. None of these dollars have been allocated for organ donation after 2007. This would mean this unique program which has made a national contribution to the donor shortage would cease to exist after midyear 2008. Currently MOTEP exists in 11 sites. Only 5 of which are partially funded. To optimize this unique community grass roots education program, funding for 15-25 sites would require 3-5 million dollars a year for an additional 5 years.

In: Organ Donation: Supply, Policies and Practices ISBN: 978-1-60692-501-0
Editor: P. T. Grinkovskiy

Chapter 3

TESTIMONY BEFORE THE UNITED STATES HOUSE OF REPRESENTATIVES, INFORMATION POLICY, CENSUS AND NATIONAL ARCHIVES SUBCOMMITTEE, OVERSIGHT AND GOVERNMENT REFORM COMMITTEE, "ORGAN DONATION: UTILIZING PUBLIC POLICY AND TECHNOLOGY TO STRENGTHEN ORGAN DONOR PROGRAMS"*

Testimony of

Jeffrey S. Crippin

American Society of Transplantation
Medical Director, Liver Transplantation Program, Barnes Jewish Hospital
Washington University School of Medicine, St. Louis, Missouri, USA

* This is an edited, excerpted and augmented edition of an Information Policy, Census, and National Archives Subcommittee Testimony dated September 25, 2007.

Tuesday, September 25, 2007

Good morning Chairman Clay, Ranking Member Turner and members of the Information, Policy, Census and National Archives Subcommittee of the Oversight and Government Reform Committee. On behalf of the American Society of Transplantation, representing the majority of our nation's professionals engaged in solid organ transplantation, we applaud your leadership for convening this forum today to focus on organ donation and our nation's ability to deliver the "The-Gift-Life" to the thousands of patients currently awaiting a life saving donor organ. My name is Dr. Jeff Crippin and I am the Immediate Past President of the American Society of Transplantation and the Medical Director of the Liver Transplant Program at Barnes Jewish Hospital in St. Louis, Missouri.

The American Society of Transplantation (AST) states in our mission statement, that we are "...an international organi2ation of transplant professionals dedicated to advancing the field of transplantation through the promotion of research, education, advocacy, and organ donation to improve patient care." Our interests and mission are very consistent with the title of today's hearing, "Utili2ing public policy and technology to strengthen organ donor programs", and we are pleased that this Subcommittee is meeting here today to discuss and examine how we can strengthen the nation's solid organ transplant system.

In addition to this hearing, the AST would like to applaud Chairman Clay (D-MO), Congressman Dave Camp (R-MI), Congressman Jim Costa (D-CA), and Congresswoman Ileana Ros-Lehtinen (R-FL) for reviving the Congressional Organ and Tissue Caucus. Your leadership in educating and raising the awareness and visibility of transplantation and the "gift-of-life" is greatly appreciated by the entire transplant community. Thank you.

The Bottom Line — Supply Does Not Meet Demand

As others have already outlined before this Subcommittee, the challenge in our field is the fact that over 97,000 individuals are currently awaiting a life-saving donor organ. Approximately 73,000 patients are awaiting a kidney, over 16,000 are awaiting a liver, 2,600 for a heart, 2,300 for a lung, and 1,600 for a pancreas. Between January and June of this year, we performed approximately 14,000 transplants with 11,083 deceased donor organs and 3,200 living donor organs.

Clearly the math is not difficult to understand why meeting patient's needs are so difficult in this environment of scarce resources. It also speaks to the fact that protecting a patient's life saving donor organ is critical. Optimal care for transplant recipients is crucial to their long-term survival. The medical problems facing the transplant patient are complex and require the attention of physicians trained in transplant medicine. However, the insurance industry often dictates the care of transplant recipients and may prevent patients from returning to a transplant center for medical management. This practice can lead to less than optimal care and, unfortunately, decreased survival rates. Furthermore, transplant centers are held accountable for the survival of their patients, even when they are prevented from delivering the appropriate care. Thus, the AST supports initiatives that guarantee longterm patient follow-up at the patients transplant center or an appropriate center within the patient's geographic region.

In an effort to protect the scarce resource of a donor organ, AST supports the following initiatives:

- Extension of coverage of immunosuppressive medications for the lifetime of the transplanted organ;
- Patient access to their transplant center;
- Access to insurance coverage, especially for pediatric patients; and
- Development of programs for patient and professionals education regarding early treatment of diseases that frequently leads to the need for organ transplants.

EDUCATION AND AWARENESS — PATIENTS & PHYSICIANS

The AST knows the education and awareness of patients and physicians alike is crucial to the delivery of effective health care. The Society has developed several educational programs to provide updated information on issues regarding organ failure and its complications, the transplant evaluation, and the transplant procedure itself. The organi2ation has crafted a program devoted to the care and maintenance of a transplant after it has occurred. Through these efforts, the AST strives to minimi2e and eliminate any questions or confusion that may arise as a patient is considering this life saving surgery before and after transplant. The Society is also actively involved in the education of physicians.

Specifically, we have a number of efforts directed at physicians not actively involved in transplant programs, but involved in the care of patients with organ failure, so a timely referral can be made to the local transplant center. The goal of these programs is to insure that all Americans have equal access to solid organ transplantation. The issue, Chairman Clay and members of the Committee are the unfortunate ignorance of those not familiar, both physicians and patients, with the criteria for transplant candidacy and outcomes. Our programs seek to address these gaps in education. That said, more needs to be done to educate the community.

In my own institution in Missouri, Dr. Amy Waterman, a social psychologist and Assistant Professor of Medicine in the Division of General Medical Sciences at Washington University, is conducting groundbreaking work examining increased patient awareness regarding kidney transplantation. Waterman is currently developing living kidney donation materials focusing on racial differences in attitudes about diabetes and organ donation. Part of her work is funded by the Health Resources & Services Administration (HRSA) through a grant looking at educating patients at kidney dialysis centers about the availability of kidney transplantation. The data obtained by Dr. Waterman and her colleagues will hopefully lay the groundwork for similar programs across America, as we continue to fight the battle against the misinformation and lack of information regarding this life saving therapy.

Outreach to Underserved Patient Populations

In an effort to reach patients in areas that remain underserved and not necessarily knowledgeable about transplantation, I have spent the last four years conducting patient outreach clinics in rural areas of my own home State of Missouri. Although my medical institution is based in St. Louis, many rural citi2ens across the State of Missouri are not able to travel to the city for education, evaluation, possible diagnosis, and treatment. To combat this situation, I and my colleagues have established clinics in underserved areas such as Cape Girardeau, MO. Cape Girardeau is a town approximately 120 miles southeast of St. Louis with a population of 70,000.

For various reasons, many of the town's citi2ens do not like to leave or travel to large urban settings and will refuse a referral to St. Louis or other large cities, in spite of a defined need. My presence and that of my colleagues has allowed these patients and their physicians to see the need for solid organ transplantation and simplified their need.

ADDRESSING DISPARITIES IN SOLID ORGAN TRANSPLANTATION

In 2002, end stage renal diseases (ESRD) Medicare (CMS) program costs $17 billion or 6.7 percent of the overall budget. In the United States, ethnic minorities suffer disproportionately from kidney diseases. African Americans comprise 35 percent of the Medicare dialysis population. Compared to Caucasians, the incidence of ESRD in African Americans in 4-fold higher than that of Caucasian counterparts. This is also true for Native Americans among Zuni Indians in the American Southwest in whom renal disease in 18-fold more prevalent than for Caucasians. Hispanic Americans have 2-fold the rate of ESRD of non-Hispanic Caucasians.

The excess burden of kidney disease in minority populations reflects, in part, the higher rate of known medical and environmental risk factors for ESRD and for other end-organ failure, including genetic predisposition, diet, lifestyle, Type II diabetes mellitus and hypertension and delays in receiving appropriate treatment. In the Native American dialysis population, 73 percent are diabetic and 83 percent are hypertensive. In African Americans, hypertension is prevalent and less well controlled by conventional medical therapies.

The Diversity and Minority Affairs Committee of the AST convened a symposium to examine organ transplantation in underserved and minority populations. The goals of the meeting included "benchmarking" of solid organ transplantation among minority populations, review of the epidemiology of the end-organ damage, exploration of barriers to transplantation services and development of approaches to eliminate disparities.

Participants in the symposium noted that minority populations were more likely to be adversely affected by limited preventive medical care, lack of counseling regarding transplant options, and delays in transplant referrals for organ transplantation. These features largely reflect economic disadvantage as well as the reduced presence of minority professionals with training in transplant-related specialties.

Participants in the conference noted that recent changes in organ allocation policies had improved access to minority individuals once listed for renal transplantation. Similar advances will be needed for other organs to address inequities in pre-transplant care and under-representation of minorities among transplant professionals. The biologic basis of differences in transplant outcomes for minority recipients has not been adequately studied. Research funds must be targeted to address biologic mechanisms underlying disparate transplant outcomes including the impacts of environment, education, poverty and lifestyle choices.

REMOVING FINANCIAL DISINCENTIVES — FAMILY AND MEDICAL LEAVE POLICIES

In 1999 the AST and other transplant organi2ations worked closely with Congress to pass and enact legislation providing up to six weeks of paid leave for federal employees seeking to donate a life saving donor organ. Congressman Elijah Cummings of Maryland spearheaded this initiative in the House of Representatives.

In addition to federal leave laws, the AST initiated its own private campaign entitled the, "AST Employee Leave and Donation Program." The purpose of this campaign is for our transplant physician members to reach out to corporate American and encourage them to amend their employee leave policies to allow adequate time for employees to serve as a living donor. This effort has resulted in many company's changing their rules and removing a financial disincentive to donation.

One of the greatest barriers at every stage of the organ transplantation process to many individuals is the lack of insurance coverage. This barrier exists from the time a prospective recipient is eligible for listing on the transplant wait list and persist after the transplant itself. Once a recipient receives an organ transplant, the AST and its membership supports measures to ensure that the care for patients are optimi2ed and that the transplanted organ will last as long as possible. To this end, a most important objective is the support of legislation providing coverage for immunosuppressive medication for the lifetime of the transplanted organ. To clarify, patients must take immunosuppressive anti-rejection medications for the life of their transplanted organ.

For many years, the federal government would pay for a transplant operation but only cover 36 months of transplant immunosuppressive drug medications. This was obviously a flawed policy that resulted in patients losing their transplanted organ, returning to dialysis in the case of kidney, or losing their life. From a pure cost perspective it also proves to be more expensive to return individuals to dialysis andIor re-transplant.

As you know Mr. Chairman, last month Congressmen Dave Camp (R-MI) introduced a bipartisan measure, H.R. 3282 to cover gaps in Medicare program coverage for immunosuppressive drugs. The legislation, the "Comprehensive

Immunosuppressive Drug Coverage for Kidney Transplant Patients Act of 2007", supported by you and other members of the Subcommittee, would be a solid step forward toward ensuring that transplant patients remain healthy.

The AST supports initiatives that ensure the coverage of immunosuppressive medications for the lifetime of a transplanted organ, regardless of age and ability to pay. Ultimately, this will lead to improved transplant success rates and the greater ability of transplanted recipients to return to a normal life.

Mr. Chairman, Ranking Member, and Members of the Subcommittee, the AST thanks you for the opportunity to participate in today's forum. We applaud and commend your leadership and efforts on this important issue.

The "gift-of-life" though often surrounded by tragic circumstances, can prolong the lives of affected Americans, allowing them to maintain their roles as active and productive citi2ens of our great nation.

In: Organ Donation: Supply, Policies and Practices ISBN: 978-1-60692-501-0
Editor: P. T. Grinkovskiy

Chapter 4

STATEMENT BY SUSAN DUNN, ASSOCIATION OF ORGAN PROCUREMENT ORGANIZATIONS, DONOR ALLIANCE, INC., BEFORE THE INFORMATION POLICY, CENSUS, AND NATIONAL SUBCOMMITTEE ARCHIVES, OVERSIGHT AND GOVERNMENT REFORM COMMITTEE, SEPTEMBER 25, 2007*

INTRODUCTION

Congressman Wm. Lacy Clay and Members of the Subcommittee,

I would like to thank you for this opportunity to testify before the Subcommittee today on the issue of saving lives and I applaud the Subcommittee for bringing these important issues before the public. My goal is to share with the Subcommittee an organ procurement organization's perspective on donation.

My name is Sue Dunn. I am the President-Elect of the Association of Organ Procurement Organizations, otherwise known as AOPO. I am also the President and CEO of Donor Alliance, Inc., the federally designated organ procurement organization (OPO) that serves the donation service area of Colorado and most of Wyoming.

---

* This is an edited, excerpted and augmented edition before the Information Policy, Census, and National Subcommittee Statement dated September 25, 2007.

AOPO represents and serves all 58 federally designated OPOs through advocacy, support, and development of activities that will maximize the availability of organs and tissues and enhance the quality, effectiveness, and integrity of the donation process. AOPO is a professional organization that is dedicated to honoring donors and their families and meeting the needs of waiting recipients by providing education, information, research, and technical assistance to OPOs, and facilitating communication and understanding among OPOs, other healthcare organizations, and federal agencies to promote the goals of organ and tissue donation.

An OPO is a not for profit organization, by statute, that is federally designated by the Department of Health and Human Services. OPOs are responsible for identification and care of organ donors and their families, organ retrieval, organ preservation, transportation, and data follow up regarding deceased organ donors. OPO staff work with donor families, and educate medical staff and the general public about organ donation.

THE CRISIS

As of September 21, 2007, just this past Friday, nearly 100,000 Americans were waiting for a life saving organ transplant. Approximately 18 of these patients die every day while waiting for an organ that never comes. The growing divide between the number of people waiting for a transplant and the number of available organs has become a national health crisis. Most organs available for transplant come from deceased donors. In 2006 there were 22,201 transplanted organs from deceased donors and 6,729 from living donors. A deceased donor may donate up to seven solid organs in addition to bone, tissue, skin and eyes which can save or improve the lives of up to 50 people. Since each donor represents the potential of saving or improving 50 lives it means that maximizing the gift from every donor, every time is of extreme importance.

EXTRAORDINARY RESULTS AND IMPROVEMENTS

A National Experiment

Since the fall of 2003, an extraordinary development has occurred as the number of donors and the number of organs transplanted reached historic record increases as well as absolute levels. The Department of Health and Human Services joined with key national leaders and practitioners from the Nation's transplantation and hospital communities in 2003 to launch the Organ Donation Breakthrough Collaborative. The Collaborative was intended to dramatically increase access to transplantable organs. The purpose of the initiative was clear, measurable, ambitious, and achievable:

> Committed to saving or enhancing thousands of lives a year by spreading known best practices to the Nation's largest hospitals to achieve organ donation rates of 75 percent or higher in these hospitals.

This major commitment by all parties focused on the sharing of accountability by all sectors to increase donation. The focus is on the application of quality improvement, team-based approaches to this important endeavor and the increased involvement of the leadership of all organizations. The results have been impressive. Clearly, the United States is far from maximizing its supply of available organs from deceased donors. In 2002, only 6,617 (about 46 percent) of an estimated 14,000 potential donors donated organs. By 2006, however, the number exceeded 8,000.

Through a case study approach, it was determined that the successful programs all had specific overarching principles and implemented effective practices that could be learned and replicated across the country to increase the number of organs available for transplantation. The Organ Donation Breakthrough Collaborative helped OPOs and their chosen large hospitals to close that gap rapidly. Multidisciplinary teams composed primarily of critical care nurses and OPO staff participated in intensive learning sessions and action periods. Participating teams achieved significantly higher organ donation rates.

AOPO's national study covering 1997-1999, published in the *New England Journal of Medicine* in 2003, documented that about 47 to 49 of every 100 medically suitable donors actually donated one or more organs. By 2006, that number had risen to around 63 to 64 percent. The national goal of 75 percent continues as a goal for all healthcare organizations.

Achieving the Collaborative's purpose of an average donation rate of 75 percent in the Nation's 200 largest hospitals saves or enhances thousands more lives each year. In 2002, the year before the Collaborative began; the number of organ donors was 6,190. In 2006 – the number of organ donors was 8,010. The first six months of 2007 show a continued upward trend for the number of organ donors on course to reach approximately 8,110 donors. (Beginning in 2004 there was a 10.8% rise in the number of organ donors as compared to the previous year, in 2005, there was an additional 5.9% increase.)

Organs Recovered and Transplanted for Each Donor is Also Critical

The number of organ donors is obviously important but so is the number of organs that are transplanted per donor. To increase those numbers, a second National experiment, the Organ Transplantation Breakthrough Collaborative was launched. Based on the same principles as the earlier experiment, this program involved members of transplant centers, donor hospitals, and the OPOs to form their multidisciplinary teams.

The teams focused on the effective practices of high performing transplant centers and began to share and implement those across the country. From 1999 through 2002, the average number of transplants per month was 1,616. In 2004 that number rose to 1,825 and continued its rise in 2005 and 2006 (1,940 and 2,039, respectively). Focusing on the 2006 numbers as compared to the 2002 numbers it is apparent that the number of lives saved increased substantially. Over the course of the year, greater than 5,000 additional lives were saved due to the increase in number of organs transplanted.

This gain, however, has occurred because of the huge increase in donors, unfortunately not matched to date by a corollary increase in the number of organs recovered and transplanted per donor. The challenge continues.

The 2006 Revised Uniform Anatomical Gift Act (UAGA)

With the organ donation crisis continuing to grow, AOPO undertook a review of the anatomical gift laws of fifty-four different jurisdictions, all of which had in place the original 1968 UAGA or its 1987 revision. The findings were striking as the Association found that there were many issues with the existing state laws:

- The anatomical gift laws were not uniform.
- The 1968 and 1987 versions of the UAGA failed to address the roles of OPOs. Since the late 1980s, OPOs have administered the process of assessing and obtaining authorization for anatomical gifts. The OPOs,

under federal law, are also responsible for assuring that anatomical gifts are properly managed, recovered, and allocated according to the national waiting list that is maintained by the federally mandated OPTN.

- There was no standard definition of a donor registry, and no core requirements for their establishment or function.
- Healthcare agents or proxy holders under a durable healthcare power of attorney were not entitled to authorize post-mortem organ donation under the 1968 and 1987 UAGAs.
- The 1987 UAGA explicitly provides that no other person may revoke a document of gift and that the assent of no other person is required for a gift to be valid. Although this was explicit in the 1987 language, some OPOs and hospitals had failed to follow the existing law so AOPO and others sought stronger and more clearly defined language to reinforce the intent of the document of gift.

After fully defining the issues with the existing laws, AOPO approached the National Conference of Commissioners on Uniform State Laws (NCCUSL) to see if it would be willing to work on another revision. As Howard J. Swibel, President of NCCUSL, stated, "Rarely do we as virtual legislators have the opportunity to literally save people's lives. This is such an opportunity, and we must seize it in earnest, since thousands are waiting for life-saving organ transplants."

The revised UAGA represents a significant, far reaching event. It is important to note that it relates only to deceased donors. Like prior versions, the centerpiece of the 2006 UAGA is the concept of "first-person" consent, under which no other person can alter the individual's decision to donate. The 2006 UAGA expressly bars a person from "making, amending, or revoking" an anatomical gift if that was the donor's wish.

The 2006 UAGA facilitates donation by expanding the list of individuals who may make an anatomical gift on a donor's behalf both during the donor's life and thereafter. The Act also expressly provides for the making of an anatomical gift on a donor registry, in addition to donor cards and driver's licenses. In time, donor registries may become the primary way people choose to make their anatomical gift known. The Act allows for the appropriate state agency to establish, or contract for the establishment of, a donor registry. It also sets forth three criteria for a well designed donor registry:

- The registry will allow a donor or other authorized person to make a gift on the registry by way of statement or symbol,

- The registry is accessible to all OPOs to determine whether an individual at or near death has made, amended, or revoked an anatomical gift,
- The registry must be accessible to donors, authorized persons acting on their behalf, and OPOs on a 24/7 basis.

If a decedent dies without having made an anatomical gift during life, the 2006 UAGA provides that a gift can be made on the decedent's behalf by his or her spouse, adult children, parents, adult siblings, grandparents, decedent's adult grandchildren, the individual who was acting as the decedent's agent under power of attorney at the time of death, and as well as any adult who exhibited special care and concern for the decedent. If none of these people are available, the gift may be made by the person having the authority to dispose of the body of the decedent (i.e., coroner, medical examiner, hospital administrator, or government official).

Under the 2006 UAGA, any member of a class (such as all of the adult children of a decedent) may make a gift if he or she is unaware of any objections by other members of the class. If an objection is known, then the gift can only be made by a majority of the class members. The 2006 UAGA also prioritizes the anatomical gift's purpose (transplantation, therapy, research, or education).

In general, the 2006 UAGA incorporates a number of important new features that will increase organ, tissue and eye donation. The 2006 UAGA can play a major role in meeting the needs of those waiting for a life saving organ but only if all the state legislatures adopt the new language. As of September 21, 2007, the 2006 UAGA had been adopted by twenty states and legislation is pending in at least eight other states. Our Association and its members continue to work hard across the Nation in achieving broad Sate acceptance and incorporation of this important set of model legislative provisions.

DonorNet 2007

Since inception of the OPTN in 1986, OPOs, transplant centers and histocompatibility labs have relied upon the telephone and the fax machine to make and review organ offers, collect and assess donor data and labs results, and ultimately accept or refuse a limited supply of transplantable organs. This voice and paper-based, work-intensive process performed repetitively and usually under great pressure had allowed for some inaccuracies, miscommunications and human errors.

Patient safety, efficiency, accuracy and equity were foremost in the minds of those dedicated to the redesign of DonorNet and the implementation of an electronic organ placement system for the Nation. The new system allows transplant centers to quickly indicate to the OPO whether they *are* or *are not* interested in accepting the organ, so that the OPO coordinator's time can be dedicated to communicating with those centers that *are* interested.

DonorNet 2007 supports a central electronic environment that enables OPOs to make multiple, simultaneous organ offers according to policy, and provides qualifying transplant centers equal and immediate access to uniform donor data and lab results. The new system became available to the community in the fall of 2006 and became fully implemented in January 2007.

To ensure that OPOs and transplant centers' needs and concerns were addressed in the design and roll-out of the new system, the OPTN/UNOS Operations Committee established the Electronic Organ Placement Working Group, whose members include physicians and surgeons, organ and transplant coordinators and administrators from a variety of transplant centers, organ procurement organizations and histocompatibility labs, as well as representatives of the AST, ASTS, AOPO and NATCO.

The involvement of OPOs in support of the development and implementation of this major information technology has been critical. The bottom line effect has already been seen in reductions in the placement time for life saving organs.

Organ Donation and Recovery Improvement Act

Congress has the unique opportunity to assist in addressing financial disincentives to living organ donation, better coordinating organ donation in hospitals, and improving the science of donation. We ask you to support an initial appropriation of $2 million for Public Law 108-2 16 which is in the FY 2008 Labor, Health and Human Services, and Education appropriations bill. The law was signed in 2004 and was authorized for five years. The legislation is in the fourth year of its five year authorization. This is the last opportunity to obtain funding for implementation of the critical programs that can save lives.

As you may know, an increase in donor organs not only saves lives, but also saves the federal government millions of dollars in dialysis and other health care costs. In the case of living kidney donation, Medicare would avoid direct dialysis costs exceeding $55,000 per year for each patient transplanted.

The need for funding this year is more critical than ever. The Division of Transplantation has received cuts or level funding for the past four fiscal years. These cuts are in spite of the Office of Management and Budget's goal of doubling the number of transplanted organs by 2013. We share the opinion, along with many in Congress and the Administration, that enactment of the Organ Donation and Recovery Improvement Act of 2004 was a very positive step toward meeting the needs of people waiting for a transplant. But, only with adequate appropriations will this bipartisan legislation allow the federal government, states, and other public and private entities to expand their current organ donation efforts and create new, effective organ donation programs.

CONCLUSION

Organ donation has seen an amazing increase over the past number of years. The spectacular force of positive action has been created by bringing together professionals from the OPOs, the donor hospitals, and the transplant centers. Other positive steps have been taken through legislative and policy efforts as well as improvements in the use of technology. The focus remains on the donor, the donor family and honoring their wishes. With the continued support of Congress, the Federal government and the stakeholders, we will be successful in saving more lives through donation and transplantation.

I would like to thank the Subcommittee for the opportunity to present the organ procurement organization perspective on the topic at hand and will look forward to answering any questions you have.

In: Organ Donation: Supply, Policies and Practices ISBN: 978-1-60692-501-0
Editor: P. T. Grinkovskiy © 2009 Nova Science Publishers, Inc.

Chapter 5

TESTIMONY OF ELIZABETH M.P. RUBIN, BEFORE THE INFORMATION POLICY, CENSUS AND NATIONAL ARCHIVES SUBCOMMITTEE OF THE HOUSE OF REPRESENTATIVES ON OVERSIGHT AND GOVERNMENT REFORM COMMITTEE, SEPTEMBER 25, 2007*

Good afternoon. My name is Elizabeth Rubin and I am here to represent transplant recipients and patient advocacy groups. To start out, I just want to tell you how glad I am to be here, or for that matter, anywhere! Were it not for the miracle of transplantation, I would have gone to the "Great Beyond" over 15 years ago, at the age of 36 years old. Up until the time I learned that my liver was failing and that I would need a liver transplant, I thought I was in tip-top shape, enjoying life to its fullest and taking my good health for granted. And, even after I had been informed that I was ill, I ignored the diagnosis and continued to pursue all of the activities that were part of my life at that time. I had just had a second daughter, and I had a four year old as well. My husband and I lived a comfortable life in the suburbs of Philadelphia, where he was employed as a business manager for an oil company, and I was working part-time as a legal assistant for a major law firm in the city. When my gastroenterologist gave me what he could of a

* This is an edited, excerpted and augmented edition of Testimony before the Information Policy, Census and National Archives Subcommittee dated September 25, 2007.

diagnosis — he couldn't really determine what exactly was wrong because all of the tests for hepatitis and known liver diseases came back negative — I did not take it seriously; in fact, I denied it, and continued to swim 100 laps every day, and, as I said, do everything else as usual. Finally, my gastroenterologist had to call my husband and tell him just how seriously ill I was, adding, "you need to get her to a hospital that can handle this, like Pittsburgh, immediately". So, we did, and within five days, I was listed for a liver transplant, entering into that cavern of the unknown, because in those days, there wasn't that much published information on what to expect while waiting or going through a transplant. I spent close to five months in Pittsburgh, four of them in and out of the hospital, waiting a total of seven weeks for a transplant and spending the remainder of the time trying to get my body to accept the foreign organ.

A lot has changed since then. Fifteen years ago, there were not very many hospitals that did transplants, and the surgery was still considered to be risky. The results were quite depressing to look at: although the percentages varied depending on the organ transplanted, many patients did not even survive the first year, and the percentage of those surviving five years was not much more. Some patients didn't make it because the original disease they had attacked their transplanted organ; others were not as good at following their post-transplant instructions; and still others could not reach the point where their immune systems accepted the 'foreign' organ. Immunosuppressive drugs were still in their infancy: the options were cyclosporine and Prograf, or FK506, as it was first called, which was still in experimental form (not approved by the FDA). In fact, those patients who were given the latter were the test cases. As I invent through the transplant process, I felt a little like an explorer breaking new grounds: I ignored the statistics, and decided that if I followed doctors' orders and took charge of my life, I would be able to break all of the records and live a long life, despite this hiccup. After all, the diagnosis that I was finally given for my liver failure was Cryptogenic Cirrhosis, which had no real cause and therefore should not repeat itself in my system. But there were some complications along the way, and it was not until my fourth year post-transplant that things started to level off and I could finally rest a little easier. Talk about a lesson in mortality!

When I was listed for transplant, there were approximately 30,000 patients on the transplant waiting list; now there are over 97,292. [LINOS as of 9/24/07] This is both a positive and a negative sign of what has occurred in the transplant world: positive, because improvements in medical technology have made it possible for more patients to be listed for transplant, but negative because the number of donors has not increased at the same pace as the number of candidates. What has been done to encourage people to donate has been quite successful: for example, the increase in donor awareness and education activities has publicized the subject of organ and tissue donation, and we can assume that it has helped convince people to sign up to be organ and tissue donors. I am a firm believer in the power of speech, and like many other transplant recipients, I spend a lot of time telling people about my transplant experience and explaining why they should seriously consider signing up to be organ donors. Other efforts to increase the number of donors include the broadening of regulations allowing individuals to become donors, the development of state registries at such places as drivers license centers, and the establishment of living donor programs. But none of these efforts have done enough: the number of organ donors is not keeping pace with the number of patients on the waiting list.

This is the topic for discussion at this oversight hearing before the Subcommittee on Information Policy, Census, and National Archives. Although it is important to review what has been done to strengthen organ donor programs, it is crucial for us to spend our time today discussing what can and must still be done to improve the system. I am honored to have been asked to appear before you. As a member of the Board of Directors of TRIO (Transplant Recipients international Organization), including past president, and as a transplant recipient myself, I feel as though I represent the heart of the transplant community. For those of you not familiar with TRIO, we are a non-profit international organization committed to improving the quality of lives touched by the miracle of transplantation through support, advocacy, education and awareness. TRIO has been in existence for over twenty years. Our goal is to help individuals who are suddenly thrust into the world of transplantation, as patients, potential donors, and/or friends or family of patients or donors, so that they may learn to navigate the system and subsequently work with others to advocate for the rights of the transplant patient. Although some of our members are candidates for transplant or newly transplanted, many are individuals who have been 'out' for an extended period of time. We are proof that "Transplantation Works"! Some of our members have had their transplants for over 15 years, and they are still living quality lives. Most of our members come to us through our website or through word of mouth, although we do speak to patients in waiting rooms and put brochures in medical offices and other locations where potential members may appear. Our members do a lot of grass roots work, getting out the word of organ donation into their home territories and intoitheir larger communities as well. Some of them work with their OPO's, and many of them work within local TRIO chapters organizing educational seminars, donor celebrations — both living and anatomical -, and participate in athletic events such as the U.S. and International Transplant Games. All of these activities raise awareness of the success of transplantation and the need for more organ and tissue donors. In addition, some of our members have gone beyond their communities to join UNOS patient committees, and one of our members is currently serving on the Transplant Roundtable. We are constantly looking for opportunities to spread the word of organ donation and to improve the public face of transplant. We know how important it is to present a positive and accurate story on transplantation: what is presented in the media definitely has an impact on the decision to donate or not. TRIO has recently taken on the task of monitoring media presentations on the subject of organ and tissue donation in advertising, film and TV production by joining a group called Donate Life Hollywood.

The efforts of TRIO members and other patient advocacy groups over the past decade have improved the rate of donation. However, they have not done enough to stem the shortage. The increase in the OPTN waiting list of transplant candidates far exceeds the increase in donor numbers every year. We are at a crossroads in the world of transplantation: the technology exists to make it possible for many illnesses to be treated by a transplant, and technology has also made the decision to donate and the carrying out of those wishes simple and straight forward.

The following are my suggestions for how we should tackle the organ donor shortage. For anatomical donors, there are five areas in which I recommend we concentrate our efforts. First of all, we should continue to expand the criteria for viable donation. We have already expanded the age range — when I was transplanted, the cut-off age was 70 — but we also need to continue the research necessary to determine what other categories of potential donors may be acceptable. Perhaps we should push for the use of "extended donors" and cardiac death to be totally accepted.

Secondly, we should push for individual registration with state registries in all states of this country. It has already been proven that the number of donors has increased in the states where registries exist, but not all states have passed laws in favor of these registries. This should become a nationwide practice and maybe there should even be a national database so that when you are traveling all OPOs in the country could know your wishes even outside of your home state where today you might be registered (today, only the region's OPO can access their own state registry if it is even in place). Furthermore, I recommend that individual registries override family objections to donation, that they be considered legal contracts, just like voter registration.

In addition, regulations need to be standardized across the United States with regard to the integration of organ donation responsibilities among hospital staff, OPOs and state registries so that viable organs are not wasted and organ procurement outcomes improve. The Organ Donation Breakthrough Collaborative has already proven that this will increase the percentage of organ donors. As stated in the Memorandum prepared for this Hearing, "During the program's first year, the 95 hospitals participating in the Collaborative achieved a 14.1% increase in donation, as compared to an 8.3% increase in donation at non-Collaborative hospitals." [page 41

Another recommendation is that we seriously examine the possibility of Presumed Consent as a law of the land. Today there are enough countries using this approach to provide the data to determine whether this would be feasible in the U.S. If it is deemed possible, then there would be a need to enlist technology to allow for online opting out using a national data base as the security to assure people that their organs would not be taken if they did not want them donated. If Presumed Consent is not deemed feasible in this country, then we should dedicate some time and funding to finding acceptable methods of offering incentives to people who are considering signing up to be organ donors.

Finally, I suggest that more effort and funding be put into educating the public on the need and reasonableness of organ donation, perhaps even rewarding organizations that do this, with grant money and formal acknowledgement of their efforts. We have already seen the Internet as a major force for general education. The UNOS web site as it is continually evolving is an excellent example of technology's use to provide public access to a wealth of information and reports that both patients and the general public need to make such decisions about donation and in choosing health care providers for transplantation. In addition, education in the form of 'advertising' is evident in today's grass roots initiatives driven by desperate families using websites and billboards to seek a donation of organs to save their loved ones' lives, but we could eliminate the controversy of individuals doing that and make it a full public press to benefit all patients, leveling the playing field as today's UNOS registry process does already in the area of listing patients.

For living donors, I have a few recommendations. In cases where living donation is possible, usually involving kidneys and partial livers, such donations are considered to be preferable to deceased donor organs due to the viability of the organ being donated. In many cases, these donor organs come from relatives who are more likely to be biologically compatible to the recipients. Occasionally, a relative comes forward who is willing to donate but is incompatible with the transplant candidate. Among new programs aimed at increasing the use of living organs to decrease the organ shortage, some OPTN members have established directed donation programs for the donation of kidneys in these circumstances. There are two such directed donation programs now: the "list" or "paired" programs. These two programs have been found to be quite successful in that they make use of more offered and therefore available organs. In the "list" program, a willing kidney donor who is incompatible with the transplant candidate he had intended to donate to will donate to another candidate from the waiting list with whom he is compatible. Meanwhile, his intended recipient will then be granted priority on the waiting list when a kidney that is compatible becomes available. In the "paired" program, two living donors deemed incompatible with their intended beneficiaries will be matched up with patients in which both donors are compatible, thereby providing each patient with a new organ. These two programs should be universally accepted at all transplant centers; regulations should be established and followed, thus removing the question of preferential treatment.

Another suggestion for living donors is to offer each and every one of them a certain amount of health and life insurance. I would also recommend that, as part of the follow-up, living donors be treated to long-term care. Even though transplant surgery has become less risky, signing up to be a living donor still requires one to go through unnecessary surgery, which may cause problems during or after the surgery.

I would like to add one more recommendation, which, although it may not directly impact upon the number of organ donors, would impact upon the longevity of the lives of transplant recipients. For years, we have been advocating for lifetime immunosuppressive coverage. It is time to push through the bill promoting this in Congress! It is economically short-sighted to be pushing for improvements in the U.S. organ donor program, if we are not also concerned with the fact that transplant recipients are dying because they cannot afford to pay for their transplant medications once their 18/36 month coverage runs out. If they don't die, they may be fortunate to receive a second transplant, which is also stupid when there is already such a shortage of organs.

I congratulate this committee for scheduling this hearing to discuss potential opportunities to strengthen and improve our nation's organ donor programs and awareness activities. I am honored to have been invited, and I hope that some of my recommendations will be considered. I hope that discussions such as these will continue, so that those of us living in the world of transplantation can help to continually update and improve the procedures and regulations by which transplant candidates live or die.

Finally, I hope all of those involved with this hearing will sign up to become organ donors if you have not already done so, and tell your family!

Thank you.

In: Organ Donation: Supply, Policies and Practices ISBN: 978-1-60692-501-0
Editor: P. T. Grinkovskiy

Chapter 6

Information Policy, Census, and National Archives Subcommittee Oversight and Government Reform Committee, "Utilizing Public Policy and Technology to Strengthen Organ Donor Programs,"*

Statement of

Timothy L. Pruett
Strickler Family Professor of Transplantation and Surgery,
University of Virginia and President Organ Procurement
and Transplantation Network/United Network for Organ Sharing

My name is Timothy Pruett. I am the Strickler Family Professor of Transplantation and Surgery at the University of Virginia and the current President of the Organ Procurement and Transplantation Network/United Network for Organ Sharing. UNOS is the nonprofit organization which operates the OPTN by contract with HRSA. It is not my intent to speak as an official representative of the transplant community, but rather for the patients and families that I have seen as an individual providing transplantation care for over 20 years.

For the most part, people of all ages with end stage kidney, liver, heart and lung problems live longer and better with an organ transplant than with other forms of medical support. Unfortunately, the numbers of people waiting for organs greatly outstrips the organ availability from deceased individuals. Because of an increasing wait time and the continuing gap between the numbers of people waiting and organs available, a number of Americans step forward each year to donate an organ to another person. Although many types of organs can be transplanted with live organs, this act of amazing generosity is most frequent for those that need and receive kidney transplants. From a system operations perspective, a kidney from a live donor is best: it lasts longer in the recipient, it is an easier operation to plan for the recipient and the medical center and it functions more quickly and reliably than one from a deceased donor. In short, if you needed a kidney, you would want to receive one from someone that was alive and not dead.

The first kidney transplant ever performed came from a live donor. In 2006, over 30% of the kidneys transplanted in the US came from live organ donors. It is a form of organ donation that our people have embraced for 60 years. The executive and legislative branches of the government have recently weighed in regarding the value of live organ donation. Because there are many instances where Americans are willing to donate, but biology gets in the way, a variety of methods of "paired donation" have been proposed to increase this type of organ transplantation. Congress has recently addressed the issue through legislation and is on the verge of passing H.R. 710, the bill named for former Representative Charlie Norwood. That bill officially provides what the Department of Justice has recently approved in memo form: that paired donation between live donors and recipients does not constitute valuable consideration and is therefore legal under Sec. 301 of NOTA.

In 2006, a directive was published in the Federal Register (Vol. 71, No. 116, 34946) instructing the OPTN to "develop policies regarding living organ donors and living organ recipients, including policies for the equitable allocation of living donor organs, in accordance with section 121.8 of the final rule". It is clear that the value of living organ donation and transplantation is an activity to be encouraged from the perspective of those in need of receiving organs, the medical community, those that reimburse organ transplantation and the government and oversight community.

The live donor does an extraordinary act; lying down on an operating room table, giving up a piece of oneself for another person and placing one's health and

* This is an edited, excerpted and augmented edition of an Information Policy, Census, and National Archives Subcommittee Statement, dated September 25, 2007.

safety in the hands of doctors and nurses when there will be no direct medical benefit for the person. Our society (and treasury) gets a great deal of benefit from this form of generosity.

Unfortunately, the pain of recovery from the procedure of removing a kidney (or any other organ) is often not the only form of pain that the donor suffers. Financial pain is also common. Significant financial disincentive to be an organ donor exists in the US. This comes in many forms: lost wages of the donor and family support members, temporary change in the ability to perform one's job during the recovery period, travel costs incurred during the evaluation to be a donor, potential ability to obtain and collect insurance benefits as a consequence of the donation process or in a worse case scenario, permanent disability, need for transplantation or even death.

We have no safety net for those that want to donate organs. Fortunately, kidney donation is relatively safe with a very low risk of death and minimal long-term morbidity, but there are multiple reports in the transplant and lay literature and even more personal anecdotes of significant financial hardship associated with the live organ donation process. This is particularly true for those individuals with personal incomes at the lower end of our financial earnings spectrum. Although the costs of the medical workup are covered by the recipient's payor, for the person without means, the personal savings, family or employers ability to help defray the additional expenses just don't exist.

As a society, we gain much in quality of life from the recipients and financial benefit through the acts of generosity that occur daily through live organ donation. I recently gave a talk at the International Liver Transplantation Society on the "Ethical aspects on live organ donation". During the discussion, there was unanimous agreement that live organ donation was not cost neutral for the donor in any country. Not only did the donation cost an organ (or part thereof), it usually cost some sum of monies from lost wages and out of pocket expenses. In this forum, the international community felt that we should do better.

In fact, if we can create a model that minimizes the personal cost to the live organ donor (family), we are likely to see more donors from people at the lower end of the financial spectrum step forward to donate for the benefit of their loved ones. An important point of this goal is that the projected cost of making organ donation cost neutral would not be more than the savings to the system as it costs more to keep someone on dialysis than to transplant them.

The major areas to be addressed should include:

1 health insurance/automatic Medicare eligibility in the event that the organ donor develops a medical condition requiring treatment as a consequence of the donation;
2 short term disability and life insurance to benefit the families of donors that either die or are unable to return to work after donation.
3 reimbursement for out of pocket expenses. A variety of methods could accomplish this end, but most would require authorization to assign these costs to the Medicare cost center at the transplant center.

The financial benefits of transplantation to our society are real. The media is fond of stating that there are not enough organs available in the US and that people are leaving this country to obtain organs from overseas. Within all ethical means, we need to increase the organ availability for those who would benefit from organ transplantation. Yes, we need to continue to develop new methods and systems that increase the numbers of organs from deceased donors. But a simple look at of our live donation system reveals that presently, we penalize the person that wants to donate an organ. As a society, we can and should be able to do better. The savings to the system by removing more people from dialysis makes the continuation of financial disincentive to live organ donation absolutely inexplicable.

In: Organ Donation: Supply, Policies and Practices ISBN: 978-1-60692-501-0
Editor: P. T. Grinkovskiy

Chapter 7

OPENING STATEMENT OF EVERSON WALLS, INFORMATION POLICY, CENSUS, AND NATIONAL ARCHIVES SUBCOMMITTEE, OVERSIGHT AND GOVERNMENT REFORM COMMITTEE *

Hearing on Organ Donation

Congressman Clay and ranking member Turner:

I want to thank you for giving me the opportunity to testify before your committee. I am humbled and honored to present Ron Springs' and my story to you. Ron is unable to attend this hearing in person because he is still going through rehabilitation; but he is doing well and is on the road to recovery. He sends his regards. Therefore, I am here representing both of us and our newly formed foundation—the Everson Walls and Ron Springs "Gift for Life Foundation" (www.giftforlifefoundation.org).

Chairman Clay, before I get into my formal remarks, I must thank my friend Raynard Jackson (who is seated behind me and has been advising Ron & I on many issues involving our newly formed foundation).

I never, in my wildest dreams, thought you would ask me to participate in a hearing before the U.S. House of Representatives. As if that wasn't enough, for you to introduce a bill in congress named after Ron & I—man, that's some heady

* This is an edited, excerpted and augmented edition of a CRS Report RL33902, dated May 1, 2008.

stuff. Even for someone who has played in and won a Super Bowl! So, I want to thank Raynard for introducing me to you and I look forward to working with you in the area of organ donation. Now, to my formal remarks.

Winston Churchill once stated, " To every man there comes a time when he is figuratively tapped on the shoulder and offered a chance to do a great and mighty thing, unique to him and fitted to his talents; what a tragedy if that moment finds him unprepared or unqualified for the moment that could be his finest hour."

I am not a hero, nor have I sought the spotlight since my retirement from the NFL in 1993. But, I received my tap on the shoulder in 1981 when I met Ron Springs. We were on opposite sides of the ball—me on defense as a cornerback and he on offense as a running back with the Dallas Cowboys.

Ron was a very unique athlete. He had size, speed, and the intelligence it took to become a leader on and off the field for the Dallas Cowboys. I was able to relate to Ron not just on the field, but off the field as well. Our friendship was strengthened by our family's bonding with each other.

After Ron and I both retired from the NFL, the relationship between our families became stronger. There was Ron's wife Adriene, his son Shawn (who is a current member of the Washington Redskins), daughters Ayra and Ashley. There was my wife Shreill, daughter Charis and my son Cameron There were good times all around-- during family vacations, cookouts, graduations, and Sunday dinners. It seemed as if life couldn't get any better.

Remember, I played in the NFL for thirteen years. I can say I have been associated with some of the most intelligent, respected, and talented individuals known in the world of sports..

I played with such great teams as the Cowboys in the 1980s and I was a member of Giants Super Bowl XXV championship team 1990. I realized how important teamwork was as a player and I have always tried to transfer that from on the field to off the field. I learned those lessons from playing for great coaches such as the great Eddie Robinson from Grambling State University, Tom Landry of the Dallas Cowboys, and Bill Parcels of the New York Giants. But I also learned much more from my fellow soldiers that fought in the trenches with me. Ron Springs was one of those fellow soldiers.

Ron had been diagnosed with diabetes years ago, but the disease became more acute with time. He had been placed on national transplant waiting list in 2004. His health was challenged by chronic kidney disease. There was failing eye sight, lack of circulation to his limbs, and ultimately kidney failure. One of the strongest athletes I have ever known began to show weaknesses that could not be imagined a few years earlier.

I, like most people, was very naïve about the symptoms of chronic kidney disease. I was fortunate that diabetes did not run in my family. Because of the many afflictions affecting my friend, I began to take a crash course on the subject of chronic kidney disease. I was very surprised at what I found out.

There are millions of Americans that are afflicted with chronic kidney disease, but minorities are affected disproportionately.

You have limited choices when you are afflicted with chronic kidney disease. One option is to start taking insulin, another option is to take dialysis. Dialysis is an extremely invasive procedure. In Ron Springs' case, it was more like a slow death. The process includes having all of your blood extracted from your body, filtered, and then inserted back into your body. It is not only invasive, but it is time consuming as well. Each session lasts 4-5 hours a day, and Ron Springs would endure d this procedure three times a week, for three and a half years. Unfortunately, during that time, Ron not only lost feeling in his legs, but his right foot and left toes were amputated. There is another option that is only for the fortunate, and that is to undergo a kidney transplant procedure. There are two types of kidney transplants. One is to receive the organ from a cadaver, the other, and more favorable procedure, is to receive the organ from a living donor.

Fortunately for Ron Springs, I volunteered to be his favorable option. After a barrage of tests, it turned out that I was a perfect match to become his living organ donor. On February 2 8th, Ron and I underwent a successful living organ donor transplant procedure. Because of this, Ron has no more dialysis treatments, and has a chance at a better quality of life. Although he has a long way to go, as far as rehabilitation is concerned, our lives and our families lives are much richer because of my decision to lay down my life for my fellow human being.

Finally, Congressman Clay, Ron and I established the "Gift for Life Foundation" to help us educate the public about the issue of organ donation. We want to educate the public on the need, the process, and the benefits of organ donation. There is a lot of misinformation surrounding organ donation that needs to be dealt with. Minorities, especially Blacks and Latinos, are extremely hesitant to register for organ donation. Some of it stems from religious reasons and others from some of the terrible things our government has done in the past, like the Tuskegee experiments.

N.F.L. Commissioner Roger Goodell and Dallas Cowboys owner Jerry Jones have pledged their support to us and our foundation to take our message across the country. They both have submitted letters of support to you for inclusion in the official record of this hearing. I would like to ask your continued support and personal involvement along with ranking member Congressman Michael Turner from Ohio.

We want to work closely with the Department of Health and Human Services, as well as the pharmaceutical industry to help us take our campaign nationally. Any help you can provide in meeting with these organizations would be greatly appreciated.

When I received this tap on the shoulder, what a tragedy it would have been if I was unqualified or unprepared for the moment that could be my finest hour. I thank God that I was able to give and extend the life of my dear friend, Ron Springs. Of all the success I have obtained both on and off the field, being used as a vessel of God is by far my finest hour. Thank you again for inviting me to participate in this hearing and I look forward to your questions.

In: Organ Donation: Supply, Policies and Practices ISBN: 978-1-60692-501-0
Editor: P. T. Grinkovskiy

Chapter 8

Living Organ Donation and Valuable Consideration*

Erin D. Williams[1], Bernice Reyes-Akinbileje[2] and Kathleen S. Swendiman[3]
[1] Specialist in Public Health and Bioethics
Domestic Social Policy Division
[2] Analyst in Health Resources and Services
Domestic Social Policy Division
[3] Legislative Attorney
American Law Division

Abstract

The central issue before Congress with respect to living organ donation is how to balance the needs of people seeking organs with one another, and with the needs of potential organ donors. While the majority of organs are harvested from deceased donors, an increasing number of donations are made by living donors each year. As new types of programs are developed to help encourage the practice of living donation, both legal and ethical issues may arise.

The primary federal law governing organ donation in the United States is the National Organ Transplantation Act (NOTA, P.L. 98-507). It permits

* This is an edited, excerpted and augmented edition of a United States Government Accountability Office report, dated April 2008.

living and deceased organ donation, and prohibits the sale of organs. Specifically, section 301 of NOTA prohibits the exchange of valuable consideration (money or the equivalent) for organs.

In December 2007, Congress specified in the Charlie W. Norwood Living Organ Donation Act (H.R. 710; S. 487; P.L. 110-144) that NOTA's prohibition on the exchange of valuable consideration for organs does not extend to paired organ donation (also known as paired donation, or human organ paired donation). Paired organ donation arises when two or more willing living donors are incompatible with their intended recipients, but compatible with one another's recipients. The donors give their organs to one another's intended recipients so that each recipient receives a compatible organ.

Living organ donation generally, and paired and other similar types of organ donation arrangements specifically, raise or at least touch upon a range of issues. These include some related to evolving transplantation systems, the directive that physicians do no harm, risk-benefit ratios, informed consent, type O recipients, resource allocation, parity, and the possibility of paying for organs.

Prior to the passage of P.L. 110-144, in the 110th Congress, several other measures were proposed. During the 109th Congress, S. 2306 would have clarified that for kidneys, paired donation, and another type of organ exchange known as list donation, were exempt from NOTA's prohibition on the exchange of valuable consideration for organs. The impact, if any, of P.L. 110-144 on the legality of list donation is unclear. In the 108th Congress, S. 573 IS would have exempted familial, emotional, psychological, and physical benefit from the prohibition.

This report contains background regarding how living donation is included within the larger organ donation construct, the likely impact that paired organ donation will have, and that list donation programs would have, on organ supply, the legislative history and legal interpretation of the term valuable consideration as it is defined by NOTA, and the various ethical and policy issues related to living donation, paired donation and list donation.

This report will be updated as needed.

INTRODUCTION

The issue of living organ donation is important to Congress because it represents one important set of possibilities for balancing the needs of people seeking organs with one another, and with the needs of potential organ donors. On one side of the balance, the drive to increase the supply of transplantable organs is fueled by people awaiting organ transplants. They are, in a sense, competing with one another on waiting lists for potentially life-saving scarce resources. On the other side of the balance, the drive to ensure that the transplant system is ethical and equitable precludes some mechanisms that would increase the supply of transplantable organs. Some options that have been rejected to date in the United States include paying healthy persons to donate their organs, and mandating that transplantable organs be harvested from all cadavers.

To maintain the most ideal balance for the organ transplantation system, Congress may now wish to clarify whether certain new types of living organ donation should be adopted to increase the supply of transplantable organs, or prohibited for ethical and/or equitable reasons.

Demand for Transplantable Organs

The demand for transplantable organs is outpacing the supply at an increasing rate. In the United States in 1988, there were 16,026 individuals on the waiting list for an organ transplant.[1] By 1995, the waiting list had increased almost 175%, to 43,937.[2] Since then, it has more than doubled, and as of April 22, 2008, the waiting list holds 98,915 individuals, including 75,524 people seeking kidneys.[3] Each day, on average, hospitals perform 56 organ transplants, and nearly 19 people die awaiting organs that never come.[4]

United States Organ Procurement System

In order to help ensure that organs are equitably distributed, Congress passed the National Organ Transplant Act of 1984 (NOTA).[5] NOTA authorized the Secretary of the Department of Health and Human Services (HHS) to establish the Organ Procurement Transplantation Network (OPTN), by contract. Currently, the OPTN is administered by the United Network for Organ Sharing (UNOS) under contract with the Health Resources and Services Administration of HHS. The OPTN and UNOS have established a national system for matching organs and individuals in need of organs. In addition OPTN and UNOS set policies for United States transplant centers and organ procurement organizations (OPOs).[6] The 1984 NOTA also prohibited the buying and selling of human organs by making it unlawful to exchange *valuable consideration* for human organs for use in transplantation.[7] The 1984 Act did, however, allow reasonable payments to be made to living donors for expenses relating to travel, housing, and lost wages in connection with the donation of an organ.[8]

Currently, the United States organ procurement system is composed of 58 OPOs which provide all the deceased and some living donor organs for the nation's 254 transplant centers.[9] Each OPO has a contiguous geographical service area designated by the federal government for recovering organs in all hospitals in that region.[10] Each OPO is required to be a member of and provide transplant candidate information to OPTN, which maintains the master waiting list of individuals seeking transplants in the United States.[11] OPOs may also implement regional organ allocation systems different from the national OPTN system for the purpose of increasing organ availability and/or organ quality, reducing or addressing an inequity in organ allocation/distribution unique to a local area, and/or examining a policy variation intended to benefit the allocation/distribution system overall.[12] In 1986, in order to help increase the organ supply available for transplantation, Congress passed legislation requiring virtually all hospitals to establish protocols requiring health professionals to make organ donor requests.[13]

Living Donation

In 2004 Congress passed the Organ Donation and Recovery Improvement Act,[14] the first federal law directly applicable in part to *living donors* (i.e., living people who donate an organ they can survive without, such as one of their two kidneys). Living donation is preferable for transplant recipients, because kidneys recovered from live donors typically outlast those from deceased donors.[15] The law amended the Public Health Service Act to authorize the HHS Secretary to award grants to states, transplant centers, qualified organ procurement organizations or other public or private entities to reimburse travel, subsistence, and incidental nonmedical expenses incurred by individuals toward making living organ donations.[16] The law also authorized the Secretary to establish and maintain mechanisms to evaluate the long-term effects associated with living organ donations by individuals who have served as living donors. For all types of donations, the law created and authorized funding for donor awareness programs.[17]

Government oversight of the living donation process is limited, and some OPOs have organized non-traditional programs for living donors.[18] A typical living donor program allows individuals to receive transplants from living spouses, parents, or friends who are willing to donate and are biologically compatible.

Questions have been raised about the entire process of living donation and the multitude of health, financial, and social post-operative risks that the living donor faces. (For a detailed discussion of these, see the final section of this report.) In part to help answer some of these questions, in 2007, Congress passed the Charlie W.

Norwood Living Organ Donation Act (H.R. 710; P.L. 110-144). One provision of the law requires the HHS Secretary to submit annually to the appropriate committees of Congress a report that details the progress made toward understanding the long-term health effects of living organ donation. In addition, as discussed in detail below, this law clarified that *human paired organ donation* does not violate NOTA's prohibition against the exchange of valuable consideration.[19]

Over time, Congress has considered a range of legislation aimed at encouraging the practice of living organ donation. For example, H.R. 1993 (109th) would have amended the Family and Medical Leave Act of 1993 (FMLA) to entitle employees covered by FMLA to leave in order to provide a living organ donation. A second bill, H.R. 2472 (109th), would have amended the Internal Revenue Code to allow a nonrefundable tax credit for a donation of a qualified life-saving organ for transplantation by a living donor, and amended the Public Health Service Act to provide that any such tax credit not be deemed valuable consideration for purposes of the ban against organ purchases. A third, H.R. 4753/S. 2283 (109th) , would have directed the Secretary of the Treasury to design and strike a bronze medal to be awarded to organ donors and/or their families.

Directed Living Donation and Valuable Consideration: Paired Donation and Other Types of Exchanges

As described above, in traditional living donation, a specific donor, who is biologically compatible with his or her intended recipient, donates an organ to that person. To accommodate willing living donors who are not biologically compatible with their intended recipients, some other types of directed exchanges — in which a donor specifies who is to receive his or her organ — have emerged. One is *paired donation* (also known as *paired organ donation* or *human paired organ donation*). In paired donation, two or more donors whose kidneys are incompatible with their own intended recipients, but compatible with each other's, trade donations. Each recipient receives a compatible kidney from a living donor.

P.L. 110-144 clarified that NOTA's prohibition on the exchange of valuable consideration for organs does not extend to paired donation. Prior to the passage of this law, the exchange element of paired donations triggered questions about whether such arrangements represented the exchange of valuable consideration for an organ. If so, these arrangements would have been illegal.

P.L. 110-144 contains the following definition of human paired organ donation:[20]

A An individual (referred to in this paragraph as the 'first donor') desires to make a living donation of a human organ specifically to a particular patient (referred to in this paragraph as the 'first patient'), but such donor is biologically incompatible as a donor for such patient.

B A second individual (referred to in this paragraph as the 'second donor') desires to make a living donation of a human organ specifically to a second particular patient (referred to in this paragraph as the 'second patient'), but such donor is biologically incompatible as a donor for such patient.

C Subject to subparagraph (D), the first donor is biologically compatible as a donor of a human organ for the second patient, and the second donor is biologically compatible as a donor of a human organ for the first patient.

D If there is any additional donor-patient pair as described in subparagraph (A) or (B), each donor in the group of donor-patient pairs is biologically compatible as a donor of a human organ for a patient in such group.

E All donors and patients in the group of donor- patient pairs (whether 2 pairs or more than 2 pairs) enter into a single agreement to donate and receive such human organs, respectively, according to such biological compatibility in the group.

Prior to the passage of the law, OPOs in Washington, D.C., and New England had implemented two types of programs for the exchange of kidneys.[21] One was paired donation, which was addressed in P.L. 110-114, and the other was *list donation*, which was not addressed in the law.

In a list donation exchange, a donor who is incompatible with an intended recipient makes a donation to a stranger on the waiting list. In return, the intended recipient advances on the waiting list for a deceased donor organ. While receiving a kidney from a living donor may be preferable to receiving one from a deceased donor, recipients of organs from deceased donors still have a much greater chance of survival than those who remain on dialysis.[22] (Dialysis is a mechanical process designed to partially perform kidney functions.)[23]

List donation is similar to paired donation in that it is a directed living organ donation exchange program that may facilitate increased organ donation. However, it is different in two distinct ways. First, unlike paired donation, list donation disadvantages people seeking transplants who have blood type O. (See the "Ethical and Policy Issues Related Living Organ Donation, and Paired and List Donation" section of this report for details).

Second, the effect of the passage of P.L. 110-114 on the permissibility of list donation is unclear. As was the case for paired donation prior to the enactment of the law, questions have been raised as to whether the exchange element of list donation violates NOTA's valuable consideration provision. The effect, if any, of the passage of P.L, 110-114 on the legality of list donation is explored in more detail in the "Legal Issues Relating to Valuable Consideration and Living Donation Arrangements" section of this report.

Congress has previously considered legislation to clarify that list donation is permissible for kidneys (S. 2306, 109th) . In addition, one version of the Organ Donation and Recovery Improvement Act (S. 573 IS, 108th) proposed an even broader exemption: that the definition of valuable consideration not include familial, emotional, psychological, or physical benefit to an organ donor or recipient.

This report first presents information regarding the impact of living donation programs on the organ transplantation system. It presents statistics related to the current system, and estimates the impact that paired and list donation programs would have on the supply of organs for transplantation, waiting lists, and deaths. Next, the report presents a legal analysis of NOTA's prohibition on valuable consideration as it relates to directed living donation exchange programs. The report concludes with a presentation of ethical issues involved in living donation, with a focus on paired and list donation programs.

IMPACT OF LIVING DONATION ARRANGEMENTS ON ORGAN SUPPLY

Living donation provides thousands of organs for transplantation each year. In 2005, the most recent year for which complete statistics are available, 6,903 organs were provided by living donors, which accounted for nearly a quarter of the 27,990 total organs donated (excluding hearts).[24] (See Table 1.) Over 95% of the organs donated by living donors were kidneys. All of the organs collected from kidney and other living donors were transplanted, while just under 86% of organs recovered from deceased donors were transplanted.

The amount of living organ donation has increased over time. The overall number of living organ donors has risen steadily from 2000 to 2006. (See Table 2.) Each year, as in 2005, the vast majority of organs given by living donors have been kidneys.

Table 1. Number of Organs Recovered and Transplanted from Living and Deceased Donors in the United States, 2005

	Living Donors		Deceased Donors		Total Donors
Organ Type	# Recov. (100% recovered were transplanted)	% of Total # Transp.	# Recov.	# Transp.	# Transp.
Kidney	6,569	37.2%	13,313	11,102	17,671
Pancreas	2	0.1%	2,045	1,464	1,466
Liver	323	5.1%	6,692	6,040	6,363
Intestine	7	3.9%	184	171	178
Lung	2	0.1%	2,374	2,308	2,310
All Organs	6,903	24.7%	24,608a	21,085a	27,988a

Source: United Network for Organ Sharing, based on OPTN data as of April 21, 2008, [http://www.optn.org/latestData/rptData.asp]. UNOS data are subject to change due to corrections.

[a] Totals exclude deceased heart donors: 2,220 recovered and 2,190 transplanted. Living heart transplants (domino)[25] have occurred in other years, but none in 2005.

The overall effect that mechanisms for expanding the pool of potential living organ donors, such as paired and list donation, will or might have on the available supply of various organs is difficult to measure. This is due largely to the fact that paired and list donation systems have only been implemented and tested for kidney donation, which is discussed below.

Research on Paired and List Kidney Donation Systems. The number of additional kidney transplants likely to result from a national paired and/or list kidney donation system depends on a number of things. The number of available kidneys could be increased by numerous factors — not all of which are necessarily desirable. These factors include selecting an optimal transplant system (list, paired, or combination) for the size of the population, lowering the degree of compatibility required for a transplant, increasing donor willingness to participate in list and paired donation programs, and avoiding systemic restrictions used to achieve equitable outcomes among recipients. The studies that have examined these factors are summarized below.

Table 2. Number of Organs Recovered from Living Donors in the United States, 2000-2006

Living Organ Donors	2000	2001	2002	2003	2004	2005	2006[b]
Kidney	5,494	6,038	6,240	6,473	6,647	6,569	6,434
Pancreas	7	4	1	3	0	2	1
Liver	402	522	363	322	323	323	288
Intestine	3	0	1	4	6	7	4
Lung	36	49	25	29	28	2	5
Heart	0	0	0	0	0	0	1
Total[a]	5,942	6,613	6,630	6,831	7,004	6,903	6,733

Source: United Network for Organ Sharing, based on OPTN data as of April 21, 2008, [http://www.optn.org/latestData/rptData.asp]. UNOS data are subject to change due to corrections.

[a]. Totals may be less than the sums due to patients included in multiple categories.

[b]. The data for 2006 are incomplete.

Despite the increase in organ donation, more than 6,000 individuals have died each year between 2001 and 2006 while awaiting an organ for transplant. (See Table 3.) More than half of those were awaiting kidneys.

Table 3. Reported Deaths on Waiting Lists for Selected Organs in the United States, 2000-2006

Organ	2000	2001	2002	2003	2004	2005	2006[b]
Heart	634	673	587	536	476	429	383
Intestine	25	45	53	49	54	55	53
Kidney	3,195	3,441	3,803	3,884	4,090	4,217	4,471
Liver	1,798	2,054	1,911	1,863	1,889	1,889	1,749
Lung	500	507	498	472	492	371	267
Pancreas	36	61	38	47	59	75	76
Total[a]	6,153	6,724	6,800	6,737	6,914	6,865	6,821

Source: UNOS, current as of April 21, 2008, [http://www.optn.org/latestData/rptData.asp]. UNOS data is subject to change due to corrections.

[a]. Totals may be less than the sums due to patients included in multiple categories.

[b]. The data for 2006 are incomplete.

One study generated data about the type of transplant system that is optimal for a given population size by comparing paired, list, and combination programs via computer model. The authors estimated that a pool of 3,584 donor/recipient pairs could generate 1,871 successful transplants (52%) using a combination paired/list exchange program, 1,730 (48%) using a paired program alone, and

1,330 (37%) using a list program alone.[26] The same study found that, for small populations of donor/recipient pairs (less than 100), list donation would generate more potential transplants than paired donation because list donation uses the entire deceased donor pool, while paired donation is limited to the incompatible pool.[27]

A second study investigated factors that influence donors' willingness to participate in paired and list exchange programs.[28] Willingness to make a paired or list donation appeared to be directly proportional to the likely magnitude of benefit to the intended recipient. Of 174 potential donors who had been found medically incompatible with their intended recipients, 63.8% were willing to participate in paired donation (in which the intended recipient would receive a kidney immediately from a live donor), and 37.9% were willing to participate in list donation (in which the intended recipient would be moved up the list for a kidney from a deceased donor). Willingness to make a list donation was greatest when the intended recipient would be moved to the top rather than the top 20% of the waiting list (37.9% vs. 19.0%).

A third study examined the possibility of maximizing paired donations by lowering the donor/recipient compatibility requirements.[29] By doing so, authors were able to increase the percentage of possible exchanges from 57% to 91.7% of patients in their database.[30] A number of specialized centers report success with incompatible kidney transplantation using special techniques to make the kidney more compatible with the intended recipient. The results of these types of transplants are reportedly encouraging,[31] but long-term results are not yet available, and therapy is labor intensive, requires immunosuppressives, and adds an average of $28,000 to the cost of the transplant.[32]

A fourth study estimated the impact that ethical restrictions to help ensure that people of all blood types benefit equitably from list donations would have on the number of transplants performed.[33] The authors proposed certain restrictions on list donation (and others have proposed avoiding list donation altogether) because people with blood type O may be disadvantaged by such a system. Donors with blood type O may give compatible kidneys to recipients with any blood type, but recipients with O blood type may only receive compatible kidneys from type O donors. For that reason, type O recipients, who already have the longest mean wait time on the cadaver waiting list, may have to wait an even longer time for a cadaveric kidney in a typical list donation program. The ethical dimensions of this issue are discussed further in the Ethical Issues section of this report.

Study results indicated that restrictions to benefit recipients with blood type O would decrease annually the number of additional kidneys available from list exchanges by about one-half (from a range of 844 — 2,155 additional kidneys, to a range of 414 — 1,150 additional kidneys). The study also indicated that, unless the restrictions were used, type O recipient candidates in a list exchange program would experience an increased waiting time that would translate into 15.17 deaths per year among the group.

LEGAL ISSUES RELATING TO VALUABLE CONSIDERATION AND LIVING DONATION ARRANGEMENTS

Statutory Prohibition in NOTA

As enacted, the National Organ Transplant Act of 1984 (NOTA), § 301(a), prohibited buying or selling human organs "for valuable consideration for use in human transplantation."[34] The original statute also included a criminal provision with fines of up to $50,000 and imprisonment for up to five years, or both.[35] While the statute did not define valuable consideration, it did state that the term "does not include the reasonable payments associated with the removal, transplantation, implantation, processing, preservation, quality control, and storage of a human organ or the expenses of travel, housing, and lost wages incurred by the donor of a human organ in connection with the donation of the organ."[36]

The legislative history of the 1984 NOTA did not discuss the meaning of the term valuable consideration.[37] It simply expressed Congress's intent to criminalize the buying and selling of organs for profit. For example, the Senate report accompanying S. 2048 stated that "[i]t is the sense of the Committee that individuals or organizations should not profit by the sale of human organs for transplantation."[38] The House conference report for that bill reiterated that Section 301 was directed toward monetary exchanges: "This title intends to make the buying and selling of human organs unlawful...."[39] During congressional hearings in 2003 on incentives to increase organ donations, strong objections were proffered against the use of direct monetary incentives to procure organs.[40]

Living donations of kidneys from a single biologically compatible living donor to a recipient had taken place before NOTA was enacted in 1984. Since NOTA specifically allowed certain expense payments to be provided to a living donor, it was clear that living donations were not precluded by NOTA and that single living donations did not implicate the § 301 prohibition against the exchange of valuable consideration. At the time NOTA was enacted, living donation arrangements involving multiple donors and recipients, such as paired donation and list donation, had not yet been developed as medical options. Thus, Congress did not consider such practices in enacting the prohibition on giving or receiving valuable consideration in return for human organs. In recent years, some transplantation facilities have implemented living donation programs involving multiple recipients and/or donors,[41] however other transplant facilities have hesitated to implement such multiple living donation programs because of possible legal concerns over whether such practices could be construed as violating the exchange of valuable consideration prohibition in NOTA.[42] Congress, in December, 2007, enacted P.L. 110-144, the Charlie W. Norwood Living Organ Donation Act,[43] which clarifies that "human organ paired donation" is not a human organ transfer for valuable consideration and thus does not violate NOTA.[44]

Valuable Consideration and Living Donation Arrangements

It has always been clear that living donation arrangements such as paired donation and list donation do not involve actual monetary payments to the donor or recipient. The concern that has been raised is whether the donors and recipients in multiple living donation arrangements have received valuable consideration for their promises to get something in return for specific acts. Such arrangements arguably involve some kind of bargain since there are mutual promises on both sides of the arrangement.[45] The argument has been made that where a donor trades his organ for a compatible organ for his intended beneficiary, the donor receives valuable consideration in the exchange of mutual promises to donate organs.[46] Now that Congress has clarified that paired transplants of compatible living donors and recipients do not violate NOTA's prohibition of valuable consideration in return for organ donation, issues may still be raised regarding other kinds of living donation arrangements such as list donation, because Congress clarified only the legality of paired donation arrangements.

Two legal opinions issued before Congress's recent amendment of § 301 of NOTA regarding paired donation arrangements continue to be relevant to the question of the legality of other kinds of multiple living donation arrangements, such as list donation. The Associate General Counsel to UNOS, in 2006, provided a legal analysis of the applicability of § 301 of NOTA to both paired donation and list donation arrangements, concluding that "NOTA §301 is legally and historically inapplicable to today's living donation arrangements."[47] Elaborating on the applicability of the § 301 prohibition on the exchange of valuable consideration, the UNOS legal analysis stated as follows:[48]

> "Valuable consideration" under NOTA § 301 is a monetary transfer or a transfer of valuable property between donor, recipient and/or organ broker in a sale transaction. It is not familial, emotional, psychological or physical benefit to the organ donor or recipient, all of which attach equally to the "living-related kidney transplants" in yesterday's terminology and to the multi-party intended recipient donations, paired donations and similar innovative and highly beneficial living donation arrangements of today and tomorrow. There is no "valuable consideration" under NOTA § 301 in any of these living donation arrangements. The donor receives none, the recipient gives none and none is transferred to a broker. In fact, there is no "consideration" at all in a living organ donation arrangement because the donation is a "gift"....
>
> A gift is different from a contract. A contract does not involve donative intent. "Consideration" and the mutual agreement of the parties are required to make the contract legally binding. A gift, on the other hand, involves a gratuitous transfer by the donor and no transfer of money, property or services or agreement not to exercise rights or to suffer material detriment ("consideration") by the beneficiary. For that reason, it is often said that no "consideration" is present in a gift. A promise to make a gift of an organ is not intended to be legally binding.
>
> The donation of an organ is properly considered to be a gift, rather than a contractual undertaking. As gifts, living donations may be made conditionally for a specific purpose. The condition can be construed as "consideration" only if the happening of the condition will be a benefit to the person who promises to give an organ. If, on the other hand, the happening of the condition will not benefit the promisor and is merely for the purpose of enabling the promisee to receive a gift, the condition is not "consideration." [footnotes omitted]

The Associate General Counsel's analysis concluded that, although list donation and paired donation involve more than a single set of recipients and/or donors, the condition in each case benefits the intended recipient rather than the donor. Thus, these transactions are conditional gifts and do not involve any federally prohibited exchange of valuable consideration.

In addition, pursuant to a request by the HHS General Counsel, the U.S. Department of Justice's Office of Legal Counsel (OLC) rendered an opinion in March 2007 on the legality of alternative organ donation practices under § 301 of NOTA. The HHS General Counsel requested the OLC's opinion so that the Secretary of HHS would know whether § 301 imposes a barrier to his engaging in various actions to encourage practices such as paired and list donation. The OLC concluded at that time that "paired exchanges and living donor transplants for increased priority in deceased donor allocation do not involve 'valuable consideration' and are therefore not prohibited under NOTA."[49] The OLC opinion examined relevant statutory provisions, the common law of contracts, contemporaneous state laws, and case law. While the opinion acknowledged that the common law understanding of valuable consideration was somewhat vague, the meaning derived from case law and the context of the term in the NOTA statute suggested that consideration, to be "valuable," should be pecuniary. Because § 301 is a criminal provision, "it is therefore appropriate to apply the rule of lenity in favour of a narrower reading, and thus to understand 'valuable consideration' in section 301 of the Act as referring to the buying and selling of organs for monetary gain or to organ exchanges that are otherwise commercial," and not to alternative organ donation practices such as paired and list donation.[50]

While Congress has made it clear that paired donation arrangements do not violate NOTA's prohibition against the exchange of valuable consideration for human organs, the legality under § 301 of NOTA of current list donation arrangements and of other, future multiple recipient/donor arrangements remains an open question. The two legal opinions cited above lend credence to the argument that such arrangements may not be found to involve illegal exchanges of valuable consideration for human organs. Further clarification of these issues would be helpful.

Ethical and Policy Issues Related Living Organ Donation, and Paired and List Donation

The central ethical question involved in organ transplantation is how to balance the needs of people seeking organs with one another, and with the needs of potential organ donors. This question has given rise to many issues, discussed below, including those related to evolving transplantation systems, the directive that physicians do no harm, risk-benefit ratios, informed consent, type O recipients, resource allocation, parity, and the possibility of paying for organs.

In order to help address the ethical issues, two groups have made recommendations, and a third has held deliberations. First, the ACOT[51] has made a series of recommendations to the Secretary. Second, the Institute of Medicine (IOM) issued a report in 2006, Organ Donation: Opportunities for Action.[52] Third, the President's Council on Bioethics (PCBE), which was created in 2001 to advise the President on bioethical issues, took up the issue of organ transplantation in its June 2006 and February 2007 meetings.[53] Relevant recommendations and discussions from ACOT, IOM, PCBE and a variety of articles are summarized in the following sections.

Evolving Transplantation Systems

As new transplantation systems test the boundaries of old regulations, the primary question arises — does Congress want to maintain direct control over key components of the system to help ensure that ethical boundaries are not breached, or does Congress want to delegate more of its authority in order to make the system more flexible?

Current law permits and defines paired organ donation (P.L. 110-144) and is, in various instances, both more and less broad than earlier proposals that were made. It is broader in that it allows paired donations for many types of organs, while many earlier proposals were restricted to kidneys (H.R. 710 EH and S. 487, 110th). It is less broad in that it exempts paired but not list donation from the prohibition of exchange of valuable consideration (S. 2306, 109th), it does not specifically enable the Secretary to determine that other similar practices are also exempt (H.R. 710 EAS, 110th), and it does not exempt the broader category of familial, emotional, psychological, or physical benefits (S. 573 IS, 108th).

ACOT proposed one possible alternative that would enable more flexibility for developing transplantation systems. The Committee recommended that the HHS Secretary seek the authority from Congress to promulgate regulations clarifying the scope of the term valuable consideration, thus allowing for the regulations' revision as transplantation technologies and methods evolve.[54] This would allow the Secretary to make modifications as new systems are developed and to develop any definitions necessary to interpret the regulations.

Ethical Issues Related to Living Donation

In medical practice generally, three primary guiding principles are that a physician should, above all, do no harm to a patient, that a procedure's benefits to a patient should outweigh its risks, and that one must obtain informed consent prior to medical procedures. The practice of obtaining organs from living donors challenges all three of these principles. Because P.L. 110-114 will presumably expand the practice of living organ donation, it raises issues with respect to these three principles, but not to a greater extent than such issues already raised by the current practice of living organ donation.

Above All, Do No Harm

The traditional first rule of medicine — above all, do no harm — would seem on its face to proscribe the practice of removing a heathy organ from a healthy person, making one a patient solely to benefit another person who is already a patient. Indeed, one survey of 100 liver transplant surgeons found that 77% experienced a moral dilemma in placing a living donor at risk.[55] Still, 72% also agreed that transplant centers had a duty to offer their patients the possibility of transplantation using living donors. IOM considered this point in its report, and suggested that the Health Resources and Services Administration (HRSA) conduct a long and full review of living donation.[56]

Risk-Benefit Ratios

The IOM also noted difficulties with living donation and the principle that a doctor should not perform a procedure unless the potential benefits outweigh the risks.[57] This calculation is generally made for each patient independently — it is not ethically acceptable for one patient to bear all of the risks and another to reap all of the benefits. On this point, IOM noted that a living donor may gain psychosocial benefits from donating an organ to one in need, which could arguably outweigh the risks to the donor's physical health. However, in order to help ensure that the risk is not too great for a particular donor due to a preexisting medical condition or the like, IOM recommended that an independent donor advocate be appointed to assess the risk-benefit ratio.

Even with a donor advocate to make the risk-benefit assessments, one major factor complicates the assessment of the ratio: little is known about the long term health and quality-of-life effects of being a living organ donor. This lack of information makes it difficult for professionals to ensure that they consider the full spectrum of risks to be outweighed by benefits. Therefore, IOM recommended (as ACOT had before[58]) that living donor registries be established to enable follow-up research on the long-term effects of living donation.[59] In addition, in June 2006, HHS solicited public comments from the organ transplant community for living donation after "several widely publicized living donor deaths" and an increasing trend in the number of living donations.[60]

Informed Consent

Ethically justifiable living organ donation presupposes the competent donor's voluntary informed consent. ACOT specified that living donors' informed consent must be competent, free from coercion, and fully informed of the risks and benefits as a donor, among other things.[61] As IOM noted, obtaining informed consent is confounded by the same lack of long-term health data that makes assessing the risk-benefit ratios difficult.[62] It is not possible to fully inform potential living donors (a necessary component of informed consent) without information about the likely impact of the procedure on long-term health. IOM suggested that creating a living donor registry would enhance informed consent as well as inform the risk-benefit analysis. Further problems in obtaining informed consent are related to the requirement that it be given voluntarily. Establishing a voluntary process may be complicated if donors are not legally competent to consent (e.g., children), or if situations are coercive (e.g., loved ones feel pressured to become living donors). Some potential donors have expressed relief at discovering that they were incompatible with their intended recipients. Expanded use of paired exchanges, and the prospect of list exchanges, may eliminate the incompatibility excuse for potential donors, and may thus create a coercive situation. IOM's recommendation that each living donor receive an advocate is aimed at protecting voluntary informed consent as well as evaluating the risk-benefit ratio. In addition, IOM recommends that the advocates address gender disparities in living donation. Women represent 56% to 59% of living kidney donors each year, and one study suggests that this is due primarily to the fact that women are asked to donate more often than men.[63]

Ethical Issues Related to List Donation: Blood Type O

Approximately 46% of the population has the blood type O, yet they represent 51.9% of people awaiting organ transplants, and 52.5% of people awaiting kidney transplants.[64] More than half have to wait more than five years for an organ (53.2%) or kidney (54.8%). No other blood type comes close to rivaling these waiting times. The percentage of people who have to wait more than five years is as follows:

- for blood type A — 28.3% for organs, and 22.8% for kidneys,
- for blood type B — 16.1% for organs, and 20.2% for kidneys, and
- for blood type AB — no recipients have to wait more than five years.

As noted previously, several authors have expressed concern that individuals with the blood type O, an already disadvantaged population in the transplantation system, may be further disadvantaged by a list donation system. Implementing a system with a disparate impact, particularly one that falls on an already disadvantaged group, has caused some authors to recommend that list paired donation have a minimal role on a national level.[65] It has caused others to recommend that the system be modified to protect type O recipients.[66]

A different set of authors has come out in favor of the list exchange program despite the impact on people with type O blood.[67] They claim that the impact on type O recipients would be transient. Though some people would be bumped to the top of the transplant list, their absence from that list when they would have come to its top (4-5 years later) would eventually balance out the impact of the system.

Current law avoids the type O issue by focusing only on paired, and not list, donation. Earlier proposals would have raised this issue by explicitly permitting list donation (e.g., S. 2306, 109th, and S. 573 IS, 108th), or potentially allowing the practice (H.R. 710 EAS, 110th).

Ethical Issues Related to Directed Donation (Paired and List)

Directed donation, which allows an organ donor to specify the recipient, creates issues related to the equitable allocation of organs. Paired and list donation (both of which are types of directed donation) create parity issues regarding what the intended recipient should be entitled to receive in lieu of the donation. Current law allows a form of directed donation (paired donation), and thus raise the issues discussed below.

Allocation

People on waiting lists for organs may wait years for a transplant, and may die before an organ becomes available. The rules governing who gets an organ are, therefore, quite important. In general, the ranking on the waiting list depends on biological matching, medical status, patient location, age of the patient, and length of time the patient has been on the waiting list for a transplant.[68] By contrast, directed donation allows the donor to choose who receives their organ (or, in the case of list donation, who is to advance on the waiting list). The PCBE noted that this raises the question of whether it is ethical for one person to receive an organ before another more needy person, simply because someone cares for them enough to make a donation.[69] PCBE also noted that prohibiting such acts of love as living donation in the name of justice would be perverse.

Parity

Some have suggested that in paired and list donations, the donated and received organs must be of equal value to ensure an equitable exchange.[70]

While this might be possible with a paired exchange, it is almost certainly not the case with a list donation, because the intended recipient will receive a kidney from a deceased donor instead of a living one. (Deceased donor organs do not typically last as long as living donor organs). Other issues related to parity have been raised, such as whether one donor in a paired exchange may change his or her mind if the other donor has already undergone surgery. To prevent these scenarios, it has been suggested that both donors should undergo surgery at the same time.[71] Other authors have suggested that outcome parity cannot be guaranteed in list and paired exchange programs.[72] If one organ fails, the recipient is not necessarily entitled to receive another.

Ethical Issues Related to Proposals for Expanding the Organ Supply: Exchanging Valuable Consideration for an Organ

The demand for transplantable organs has inspired a wide variety of proposals to increase the supply, including some that would allow or encourage forms of payment for organs. Congress has considered several proposals to give donors honorific or tax incentives for donating organs.[73] The use of financial incentives has been studied, proposed and debated in the general literature. Various organizations, including the American Medical Association and UNOS have supported the study of financial options to encourage organ donations.[74] Arguments have been made that donors of organs should be treated no differently than donors of tissues[75] (such as human hair, blood plasma, sperm, and eggs). It has also been argued that because the practice of transplanting organs is profitable for the professional parties involved, those from whose bodies the organs are harvested should be able to share in some of the profits.[76]

There has been resistance to proposals that encourage commodification of human organs. The IOM conducted an extensive analysis of various types of financial incentives to encourage donation, such as payment through regulated futures markets, payment of funeral expenses, providing bereavement counseling, tax incentives, and providing health insurance.[77] IOM concluded that none should be promoted at this time because of a lack of evidence that these incentives would improve donation rates, because once put in motion a system of financial incentives would be difficult to reverse, and because of fears that such systems might disproportionately affect the poor. This recommendation came as a disappointment to some who seek to increase the supply of transplantable organs.[78]

While current law clarifies that paired donation does not violate NOTA's prohibition on the exchange of human organs for valuable consideration, it does not permit the payment of money in exchange for organ donation. To date, Congress has not considered legislation that would do so.

References

[1] Institute of Medicine, Organ Donation: Opportunities for Action, (Washington, DC: National Academies Press, 2006) (hereinafter referred to as IOM Report), p. 19.

[2] Id. at p. 19.

[3] Data is from the United Network of Organ Sharing (UNOS) website, at [http://www.unos.org/], visited April 22, 2008. Data on the site are continuously updated. Note: In March 2008, questions were raised about the accuracy of the waiting list numbers. See Robert Stein, "A Third of Patients on Transplant Waiting List Are Not Eligible," The Washington Post, March 22, 2008, p. A01, at [http://www.washingtonpost.com/wp-dyn/content/article/2008/03/21/ AR2008032102981.html].

[4] Eric Cohen, *Organ Transplantation: Defining Ethical and Policy Issues*, President's Council on Bioethics Working Paper, June 2006 (hereinafter E.Cohen).

[5] P.L. 98-507, 42 U.S.C. 274 *et seq.*

[6] § 201 of NOTA, 42 U.S.C. § 274.

[7] § 301 of NOTA, 42 U.S.C. § 274e(a). The statute does not define valuable consideration, leading to some ambiguity in the case of living donation arrangements where mutual promises are exchanged to facilitate multiple organ donations. Even though monetary payments are not involved in such arrangements, legal issues have been raised concerning application of this prohibition against the exchange of valuable consideration. See legal discussion, *infra,* beginning on page 10.

[8] § 301(c)(2) of NOTA, 42 U.S.C. § 274e(c)(2).

[9] UNOS, Members, at [http://www.optn.org/members/], visited April 23, 2008.

[10] Howard M. Nathan et al., "Organ donation in the United States," *American Journal of Transplantation*, vol. 3, supp. 4 (2003) (hereinafter, H.M. Nathan), p. 29.

[11] All U.S. transplant centers and organ procurement organizations must be members of the OPTN to receive any funds through Medicare. § 1138 of

P.L. 99-509, the Omnibus Budget Reconciliation Act of 1986, 42 U.S.C. 1 320b-8. Other OPTN members include independent histocompatibility laboratories involved in organ transplantation; relevant medical, scientific, and professional organizations; relevant voluntary health and patient advocacy organizations; and members of the general public with a particular interest in donation and/or transplantation. Profile, About OPTN, at [http://www.optn.org/optn/profile.asp].

[12] OPTN Policy #3.1.7 (February 21, 2008), at [http://www.optn.org/ PoliciesandBylaws2/ policies/pdfs/policy_3 .pdf].

[13] § 9318(a) of P.L. 99-509, the Omnibus Budget Reconciliation Act (OBRA) of 1986, 42 U.S.C. § 1320-8.

[14] P.L. 108-216, 42 U.S.C. § 273 *et seq.*

[15] Sommer E. Gentry, Dorry L. Segev, and Robert A. Montgomery, "A Comparison of Populations Served by Kidney Paired Donation," *American Journal of Transplantation*, vol. 5, no. 8 (August 2005), (hereinafter, S. E. Gentry) p. 1914.

[16] § 3 of P.L. 108-2 16, 42 U.S.C. § 274f.

[17] § 4 of P.L. 108-216; 42 U.S.C. 274f-1. A total of $5 million was authorized to be appropriated from FY2005 through FY2009, however, the program was unfunded in FY2005.

[18] IOM Report, p. 309; H.M. Nathan, p. 39.

[19] NOTA, Section 301, 42 U.S.C. §274(e)

[20] P.L. 110-144, §2; 42 U.S.C. §274e(c)(4). This law also provides that it shall not be construed to alter or amend the Social Security Act.

[21] H.M. Nathan, p. 39.

[22] Francis L. Delmonico et al., "Donor Kidney Exchanges," *American Journal of Transplantation*, vol. 4, no. 10 (October 2004), (hereinafter, F.L. Delmonico), p. 1632.

[23] UNOS, *definition of dialysis*, at [http://www.unos.org/ resources/ glossary.asp#D].

[24] United Network for Organ Sharing, based on OPTN data as of August 3, 2007, at [http://www.optn.org/latestData/rptData.asp].

[25] A domino transplant is a procedure in which an organ is removed from one transplant candidate and immediately transplanted into a second patient, with the first patient receiving a new organ from a deceased donor. For example, lung transplants are more successful if accompanied by a donor heart as well as the lungs. A person with a healthy heart and in need of lungs might donate his or her heart if a heart/lung set became available.

[26] S. E. Gentry, 1917-1918.

[27] Id. at p. 1918.

[28] A.D. Waterman et al., "Incompatible Kidney Donor Candidates' Willingness to Participate in Donor-Exchange and Non-directed Donation," American Journal of Transplantation, vol. 6, no. 7 (July 2006), p. 1631.

[29] Requirements for human leukocyte antigen matching (HLA) were lowered from four points of compatibility to three.

[30] Inessa Kaplan et al., "A Computer Match Program for Paired and Unconventional Kidney Exchanges," American Journal of Transplantation, vol. 5, no. 9 (September 2005), p. 2308.

[31] For example, see Robert A. Montgomery et al., Clinical Results From Transplanting Incompatible Live Kidney Donor/Recipient Pairs Using Kidney Paired Donation," Journal of the American Medical Association, vol. 294, no. 13 (October 2005), p. 1655.

[32] S.E. Gentry, p. 1919.

[33] Lainine Friedman Ross and Stefanos Zenios, Restricting Living-Donor-Cadaver Donor Exchanges to Ensure that Standard Blood Type O Wait-List Candidates Benefit," Transplantation, vol. 78, no. 5 (September 15, 2004), (hereinafter, L.F. Ross), pp. 641-646.

[34] 42 U.S.C. § 274e(a).

[35] § 301(b) of NOTA, 42 U.S.C. § 274e(b).

[36] § 301(c)(2) of NOTA, 42 U.S.C. § 274e(c)(2).

[37] According to one author, the prohibition against selling organs was enacted in part because of a Virginia physician's efforts to address the organ shortage by brokering living donors' kidneys and earning a profit. Fred H. Cate, Human Organ Transplantation: The Role of Law, 20 Journal of Corporation Law, 69, at 80 (1994).

[38] See S.Rept. 98-382 (1984), at 16-17, reprinted in 1984 U.S.C.C.A.N. 3975, 3982-3983.

[39] H.Rept. 98-1127 (1984), at 16, reprinted in 1984 U.S.C.C.A.N. 3989, 3992.

[40] Assessing Initiatives to Increase Organ Donations: Hearing Before the House Subcomm. On Oversight & Investigations of the House Comm. on Energy & Commerce, 108th Cong., at 5, 21, 64-67 (2003).

[41] Johns Hopkins Medical Center began a paired organ donation program in 2001. To date, at least twenty-two patients have benefitted from the program, and, recently, the first threeway swap involving 6 people, was completed. Sarah E. Statz, Note, Finding the Winning Combination: How Blending Organ Procurement Systems Used Internationally Can Reduce the Organ Shortage, 39 Vanderbilt Journal of Transnational Law 1677, 1704 (2006).

[42] Floor statement of Senator Carl Levin on introduction of the Living Kidney Organ Donation Clarification Act, S. 2306, 109th Cong., February 17, 2006, available at [http://www.govtrack.us/congress/record.xpd?id=109-s20060216-31&person=300001], visited March 3, 2007. "Although most ethicists, lawyers and members of Congress believed that NOTA was never intended to be applied to paired organ donation, most transplant centers were persuaded against assuming they could aggressively develop such programs, even though studies claimed that the programs could generate an additional 1,550 kidney transplants every year." Bill Lawrence, For the Greater Good, UNOS Update, 22 (January-February 2008). [http://www.unos.org/SharedContentDocuments/Jan_Feb08_NotesFromHill.pdf].

[43] An UNOS Press Release regarding passage of this bill stated: "The bill honors the memory of the late Rep. Charlie Norwood of Georgia, sponsor of the bill in the House. Rep. Norwood was a lung transplant recipient and a tireless advocate for others in need of lifesaving transplantation. UNOS also wishes to thank Sen. Carl Levin of Michigan, the sponsor of the Senate bill." [http://www.unos.org/news/newsDetail.asp?id=987].

[44] P.L. 110-144 defines "human organ paired donation" in Section 2 of the Act, codified to 42 U.S.C. § 274e©). The Act also provides that the Secretary of HHS submit an annual report to Congress detailing the progress made towards understanding the long-term health effects of living organ donation.

[45] See Michael T. Morley, Note, Increasing the Supply of Organs for Transplantation Through Paired Organ Exchanges, 21 Yale Law and Policy Review, 221, 255-261 (2003).

[46] While one may find state court cases stating that "(a)ny act or promise which is of benefit to one party or disadvantage to the other is a sufficient consideration to support a contract," Steinberg v. Chicago Med. Sch., 371 N.E.2d 634, 639 (Ill. 1977), one may also find cases stating that the fulfillment of a promisor's condition that is merely for the purpose of enabling the promisee to receive a gift, does not constitute consideration for a contract. See Stelmack v. Glen Alden Coal Co., 14 A.2d 127, 128-129 (Pa. 1940).

[47] Malcolm E. Ritsch, Jr., Position Statement: Kidney Paired Donations, Kidney List Donations and NOTA § 301, at 2 (September 18, 2006).

[48] Id. at 3.

[49] Press Release, "Justice Department Finds Paired Donation Consistent with Federal Law," April 5, 2007, available at [http://www.unos.org/news/

newsDetail.asp?id=830]. This published opinion will be binding on all U.S. Attorney's offices.

[50] C. Kevin Marshall, "Memorandum for Daniel Meron, General Counsel, Department of Health and Human Services Re: Legality of Alternative Organ Donation Practices Under 42 U.S.C. § 274e," (March 28, 2007) at 6. Memorandum is available at [http://www.usdoj.gov/olc/2007/ organtransplant.pdf].

[51] ACOT was established under the authority of 42 U.S.C. Section 217a. See the ACOT website, at [http://www.organdonor.gov/research/acot.htm].

[52] IOM Report.

[53] Background materials and transcripts from the PCBE's June 2006 meeting on organ transplantation are available at the PCBE site, at [http://www.bioethics.gov/topics/ organ_index.html].

[54] ACOT, Recommendation 36, November 4-5, 2004, at [http://www.organdonor.gov/ research/acotrecssumm36-42.htm].

[55] S.J. Colter et al., "Adult living donor liver transplantation: Perspectives from 100 liver transplant surgeons," Liver Transplantation, vol 9, no. 6, pp. 637-644 (2003), in IOM Report, p. 307.

[56] IOM Report, p. 308.

[57] Id. at pp. 312-315.

[58] ACOT, Recommendation #42, May 9-10 2005, at [http://www.organdonor. gov/research/ acotrecssumm36-42.htm].

[59] IOM Report, p. 276.

[60] HHS, HRSA, Federal Register, June 16, 2006, p. 34946.

[61] ACOT, Recommendation #1, November 18-19, 2002, at [http://www.organ donor.gov/ research/acotrecsbrief.htm].

[62] IOM Report, p. 315.

[63] Id. at p. 318.

[64] The statistics in this paragraph are from UNOS, current as of February 9, 2007 [http://www.optn.org/latestData/rptData.asp].

[65] S. E. Gentry, p. 1920.

[66] L.F. Ross, pp. 641-646.

[67] F.L. Delmonico, p. 1632.

[68] For a description of the process, see, UNOS, Fact Sheets, Prioritizing patients for transplantation [http://www.unos.org/resources/FactSheets.asp].

[69] E. Cohen, p. 15.

[70] See, for example, Douglas J. Norman, "Commentary" Nature Clinical Practice- Nephrology, vol. 2, no. 6 (June 2006), p. 303.

[71] Id. at p. 303.

[72] F.L. Delmonico, p. 1633.

[73] The 107th Congress considered S. 325 and H.R. 708 (which would have given donors a Congressional medal), and H.R. 1872 and H.R. 2090 (which would have provided tax credits for donation).

[74] See testimony of Dr. Robert M. Sade, 2003 House Hearing, supra, available at [http://energycommerce.house.gov/ reparchives/108/Hearings/ 06032003 hearing946/ Sade1500.htm], visited March 3, 2007; and UNOS press release, OPTN/UNOS Board Endorses Studies of Incentives to Increase Donation (June 28, 2002), available at [http://www.unos.org/news/ newsDetail.asp?=1].

[75] Tissues, such as corneas, plasma, and gametes, are distinct from and regulated under an entirely different system than organs.

[76] See, for example, President's Council on Bioethics, "On the Body and Transplantation: Philosophical and Legal Context, Appendix: 'Organs' and 'Tissues' in the Therapeutic Transplantation Context," Staff Discussion Paper, February 15-16, 2007, pp. 2-3.

[77] IOM Report, pp. 269-302.

[78] See, for example, Richard Epstein, "Kidney Beancounters," The Wall Street Journal, May 15, 2006, p. A5.

In: Organ Donation: Supply, Policies and Practices ISBN: 978-1-60692-501-0
Editor: P. T. Grinkovskiy

Chapter 9

ORGAN TRANSPLANT PROGRAMS: FEDERAL AGENCIES HAVE ACTED TO IMPROVE OVERSIGHT, BUT IMPLEMENTATION ISSUES REMAIN*

United States Government Accountability Office

WHAT GAO FOUND

Limitations in federal oversight of organ transplant programs existed when high-profile problems came to light in 2005 and 2006. These high-profile cases included, for example, a transplant program that lacked a full-time surgeon for over a year and had been turning down organs offered for patients at markedly high rates. At that time, CMS did not actively monitor heart, liver, lung, and intestine transplant programs, relying instead primarily on complaints to detect problems. CMS periodically monitored kidney transplant programs through on-site inspections, known as surveys, but the surveys reviewed compliance with requirements that had not been substantially updated in decades and were limited in scope. In addition, some programs were not actively monitored. At the same time, the OPTN actively monitored transplant programs for many types of potential problems and worked with the programs to resolve identified problems. The OPTN's monitoring activities, however, were not

* This is an edited, excerpted and augmented edition from a GAO Report GAO-08-412, dated April 2008.

sufficient to promptly detect certain problems that prolonged the time that patients waited for transplants, such as inadequate staffing at transplant programs.

CMS, HRSA, and the OPTN have made or plan to make changes to strengthen their oversight of organ transplant programs, but the effectiveness of these changes will depend, in part, on implementation and information sharing by CMS, HRSA, and the OPTN. In 2006, after high-profile problems came to light, CMS began actively monitoring heart, liver, lung, and intestine transplant programs. In a more fundamental change, CMS published new regulations in 2007 that establish a single set of updated requirements for all Medicare- approved transplant programs and provide for periodic reviews of programs. The OPTN has been working with HRSA to develop and implement a set of indicators to better detect problems that prolong the time patients wait for transplants. However, neither CMS nor the OPTN has fully implemented these changes, and their full effect remains to be seen. In particular, CMS has not determined the extent to which it will conduct on-site surveys in its periodic reviews of programs for Medicare reapproval. Under the new regulations, CMS may choose not to conduct on-site reapproval surveys of programs meeting certain Medicare requirements. Not conducting these surveys may limit CMS's ability to monitor for compliance with other Medicare requirements and to detect problems like some of those involved in the high- profile cases. As of January 2008, CMS had not determined how it will choose which transplant programs to survey, if any, among those for which it has discretion. Further, while CMS, HRSA, and the OPTN recognize the value of sharing information about potential problems at transplant programs, how they will share additional information from their oversight activities has not been resolved. A definitive agreement between CMS and HRSA on this issue will better ensure that problems at transplant programs are detected and corrected in a timely manner.

WHY GAO DID THIS STUDY

Media reports in 2005 and 2006 highlighted serious problems at organ transplant programs, calling attention to possible deficits in federal oversight. Two agencies in the Department of Health and Human Services (HHS) oversee organ transplant programs: the Centers for Medicare & Medicaid Services (CMS) oversees transplant programs that receive Medicare reimbursement, and the Health Resources and Services Administration (HRSA) oversees the Organ Procurement and Transplantation Network (OPTN), which manages the nation's organ allocation system. GAO was asked to examine (1) federal oversight of transplant programs at the time the high-profile cases came to light in 2005 and 2006 and (2) changes that federal agencies have made or planned since then to strengthen oversight. GAO interviewed CMS, HRSA, and OPTN officials and reviewed agency documents and data and a CMS draft proposal for sharing information with HRSA.

What GAO Recommends

GAO recommends that the Secretary of Health and Human Services direct (1) CMS to develop a methodology for conducting onsite surveys for Medicare reapproval to ensure that at least some programs meeting certain Medicare criteria are surveyed and (2) CMS and HRSA to establish a time frame for finalizing an agreement to share information from their oversight activities. HHS concurred with both recommendations.

Abbreviations

CMS	Centers for Medicare & Medicaid Services
CoP	condition of participation
ESRD	end-stage renal disease
HHS	Department of Health and Human Services
HMO	health maintenance organization
HRSA	Health Resources and Services Administration
MPSC	Membership and Professional Standards Committee
NCD	national coverage determination
OPTN	Organ Procurement and Transplantation Network
UNOS	United Network for Organ Sharing

April 29, 2008

The Honorable Charles E. Grassley
Ranking Member

Committee on Finance
United States Senate

Dear Senator Grassley:

Organ transplantation has become increasingly common, with over 28,000 organ transplants performed in the United States in 2007. Over 250 U.S. hospitals have organ transplant centers. Many of these centers operate multiple transplant programs that each specialize in the transplantation of a specific organ, such as the kidneys, heart, liver, lungs, intestines, or pancreas. Despite increases in organ donations, the demand for organs continues to exceed the available supply.[1] Over 6,000 people die each year in the United States while waiting for organ transplants. The scarcity of organs relative to demand emphasizes the need to ensure both the equitable allocation of organs and proper oversight of the organ transplantation system, including the programs that perform organ transplants.

Two agencies within the Department of Health and Human Services (HHS) are involved in overseeing the organ transplantation system. These two agencies have responsibilities that differ in some respects but overlap in others.

- HHS's Health Resources and Services Administration (HRSA) is responsible for overseeing the Organ Procurement and Transplantation Network (OPTN), a nonprofit network of transplant centers and others in the transplant community that was established in 1984 to manage the nation's organ allocation system. The OPTN's responsibilities include maintaining a list of individuals waiting for transplants, operating a computerized system for matching donated organs with individuals on the waiting list, and developing policies for how organs are to be allocated. The OPTN is administered by a nonprofit organization that has a contract with HRSA.[2] Historically, the OPTN's primary focus has been ensuring the equitable allocation of donated organs, and its policies include detailed allocation rules for matching donated organs with individuals on the waiting list.[3] Its policies also address other areas related to transplantation, such as the training and experience of key transplant personnel and performance standards for transplant programs related to patient survival rates and transplant activity. More recently the OPTN's activities expanded to include monitoring members' compliance with federal regulations and OPTN policies. The OPTN monitors its members' compliance through various mechanisms, such as on-site reviews of transplant programs and regular reviews of organ allocations, and is responsible for reporting member noncompliance and any other issues affecting patient health or public safety to HRSA.
- HHS's Centers for Medicare & Medicaid Services (CMS)[4] is responsible for regulating transplant programs that receive

reimbursement under the Medicare program.[5] CMS oversees fewer transplant programs than the OPTN because not all transplant programs participate in Medicare.[6] In addition, CMS's range of requirements for Medicare-approved transplant programs differs from the OPTN's; for example, CMS does not have specific requirements for organ allocation procedures. At the same time, CMS's requirements address some areas in common with the OPTN, such as minimum qualifications for some transplant program personnel and patient survival rates. CMS has monitored some transplant programs by contracting with state agencies to conduct routine on-site inspections, known as surveys.

In 2005 and 2006, media reports of problems at several organ transplant programs drew attention to possible shortcomings in federal oversight, noting that some problems were not detected or addressed by the OPTN or CMS in a timely fashion. Three cases that occurred at different facilities in California received particular attention because of the seriousness of the problems involved. The OPTN's oversight brought one of the cases to light, while individuals alerted federal agencies or the media to the other cases.

- In 2003, a liver transplant program used one patient's high position on the waiting list to obtain a liver for someone else who was lower on the waiting list, bypassing more than 50 patients who had higher priority for the liver than the actual recipient. Medical records were falsified to conceal the switch, and the patient who had the highest priority for the liver later died without a transplant. A routine OPTN on-site review in 2005 led the transplant program's staff to review the case and self-report the problem to the OPTN.
- At another facility, the liver transplant program did not have a full-time transplant surgeon on staff even though it had led the OPTN and patients to believe otherwise. From mid-2004 until the program closed over a year later, the program lacked a full-time surgeon and had been turning down organs offered for patients on the waiting list at rates markedly higher than regional and national averages. A patient complaint in 2005 led to a CMS investigation that first uncovered the situation.
- In 2004, a health maintenance organization (HMO) notified over 1,500 of its enrollees waiting for kidney transplants that it would no longer pay for their transplants unless they were performed at a new kidney transplant program it was about to open. The new transplant program, however, was unable to properly handle the large influx of patients and did not provide contingency plans for patients to receive transplants through other programs. As a result, patients' access to transplants was impeded. A whistleblower contacted the media, and

in May 2006, media articles about the situation alerted the OPTN and CMS to the problem.

Concerned that these recent issues at organ transplant programs could indicate more systemic problems, you asked us to examine federal oversight of the organ transplantation system. This report discusses (1) federal oversight of transplant programs at the time the high-profile cases came to light in 2005 and 2006 and (2) the changes that federal agencies have made or planned since then to strengthen their capacity to detect and resolve compliance problems at organ transplant programs.[7]

Our review encompassed the OPTN's and HRSA's activities to oversee organ transplant programs and CMS's activities to oversee Medicare- approved organ transplant programs.[8] To examine the OPTN's, HRSA's, and CMS's oversight activities, we reviewed relevant laws, regulations, policies, and other documents and interviewed OPTN and HRSA officials and officials from CMS's central office and from the 5 (of 10) regional offices responsible for overseeing the largest numbers of transplant programs. We also reviewed case files from the OPTN detailing the OPTN's review of and actions taken on compliance cases that occurred from 2003 through 2006, including the three high-profile cases;[9] the OPTN's data on transplant programs that did not meet OPTN performance standards for clinical outcomes or transplant activity from January 2003 through October 2006; the OPTN contract with HRSA; CMS data on surveys of renal (kidney) transplant programs; CMS data on reviews of extra-renal (heart, liver, lung, and intestine) transplant programs conducted in 2006 and 2007;[10] CMS complaint investigations of the three high-profile cases; and a CMS draft proposal for sharing information with HRSA. We examined the reliability of the data used in this report by performing appropriate electronic data checks and checks for obvious errors, such as missing data and data outside of expected ranges. We also interviewed officials who were knowledgeable about the data. We determined that the data we used were sufficiently reliable for our purposes. In addition, we conducted interviews with experts from associations representing transplant professionals about both CMS's and the OPTN's oversight of transplant programs. We conducted this performance audit from August 2006 through April 2008 in accordance with generally accepted government auditing standards. Those standards require that we plan and perform the audit to obtain sufficient, appropriate evidence to provide a reasonable basis for our findings and conclusions based on our audit objectives. We believe that the evidence obtained provides a reasonable basis for our findings and conclusions based on our audit objectives.

RESULTS IN BRIEF

Limitations in federal oversight of organ transplant programs existed at the time high-profile problems came to light in 2005 and 2006. The nature of these limitations differed for CMS and the OPTN. CMS's oversight activities for both extra-renal and renal transplant programs were incomplete in several respects. For example, until 2006, CMS did not actively monitor extra-renal transplant programs; instead, the agency relied primarily on complaints to detect problems. CMS did periodically monitor renal transplant programs through contracts with state agencies to conduct on-site surveys and did act to resolve identified problems, but the surveys reviewed compliance with requirements that had not been substantially updated in decades and were limited in scope. In addition, some programs were not actively monitored. In contrast, the OPTN actively monitored for many types of noncompliance and poor performance and acted to resolve identified problems. The OPTN's monitoring activities, however, did not include methods capable of promptly detecting certain problems that prolonged the time that patients waited for transplants, such as insufficient staffing at transplant programs. For example, until media reports surfaced, the OPTN was not aware of such problems in two of the high-profile cases. The OPTN also did not always meet its goals for conducting on-site reviews, one component of its monitoring activities.

CMS, HRSA, and the OPTN have made or plan to make changes to strengthen federal oversight of organ transplant programs, but the effectiveness of the changes will depend in part on their implementation and the degree of information sharing that the agencies agree to undertake. In 2006, after high-profile problems came to light, CMS began actively monitoring extra-renal transplant programs. In a more fundamental change, CMS published new Medicare regulations in 2007, establishing a single set of expanded and updated requirements for both extra-renal and renal transplant programs and procedures for periodic reviews of Medicare-approved programs. For its part, the OPTN, with HRSA's involvement, has taken steps to address previous shortcomings. For example, the OPTN has been working with HRSA to develop and implement a set of indicators to better detect problems that prolong the time patients wait for transplants. The effects of CMS's and the OPTN's changes remain to be seen, however, as not all changes have been fully implemented. In particular, CMS has not determined the extent to which it will include on-site surveys in its periodic reviews of transplant programs for Medicare reapproval. Under the new regulations, CMS may choose not to conduct on-site reapproval surveys of transplant programs meeting certain Medicare requirements. Not conducting such surveys may limit CMS's ability to monitor these programs for compliance with other Medicare requirements and to detect problems like some of those involved in the high-profile cases. As of January 2008, CMS had not determined how it will choose which transplant programs to survey for reapproval, if any, among those for which it has discretion. Further, CMS and HRSA have not determined how they will share information about potential problems at transplant programs. CMS developed a proposal outlining how the agencies could share such information, but the agencies have not yet finalized an agreement. Finalizing an agreement delineating the scope and a time frame for sharing information from their oversight of transplant programs is important to ensure that in the future problems at transplant programs are detected and corrected in a timely manner.

To increase opportunities for identifying potential problems at transplant programs, we are recommending that the Secretary of Health and Human Services direct the Administrator of CMS to develop a methodology for conducting on-site surveys for Medicare reapproval to ensure that at least some transplant programs meeting certain Medicare requirements receive an on-site survey, and that the Secretary direct the Administrators of CMS and HRSA to establish a time frame for finalizing an agreement for CMS, HRSA, and the OPTN to share information from their oversight activities.

In commenting on a draft of this report, HHS concurred with our recommendations. HHS agreed that CMS should develop a methodology for conducting on-site surveys for Medicare reapproval, noting that CMS has developed an initial framework for doing so but that its implementation will depend on resources. HHS also agreed with our recommendation that HRSA and CMS establish a time frame for finalizing an agreement to share information from their oversight activities. The comments noted that CMS would like to finalize an agreement with HRSA by June 30, 2008, and that even in the absence of a formal agreement, CMS and HRSA have shared information on several occasions.

BACKGROUND

Organ transplants are becoming increasingly common. The 28,352 organ transplants performed in the United States in 2007 represent an increase of about 40 percent since 1997. (See fig. 1.) Kidney transplants are the most common procedure, accounting for almost 60 percent of transplants. Most transplanted organs come from deceased donors, but a significant portion (22 percent in 2007) come from living donors who may donate, for example, a kidney or a segment of liver or lung.

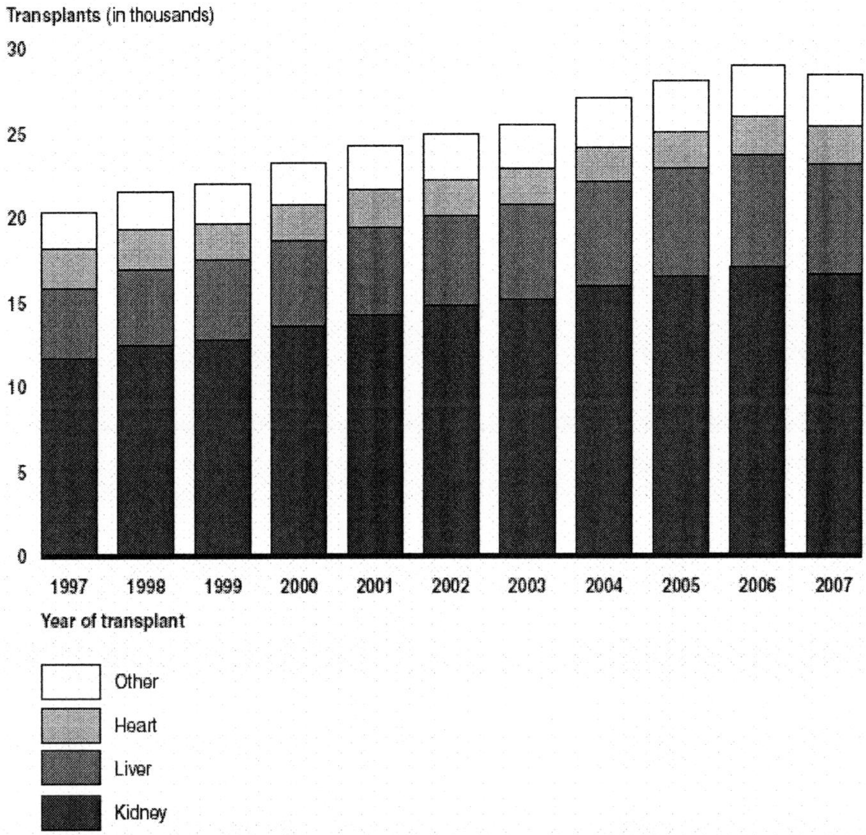

Notes: Data are as of February 29, 2008. Other includes lung, pancreas, and intestine transplants as well as procedures involving the transplantation of multiple organs, such as kidney-pancreas and heart-lung transplants.

Source: The OPTN.

Figure 1. Number of Organ Transplants Performed, Calendar Years 1997–2007.

As of January 2008, 254 U.S. hospitals had a transplant center; collectively, these centers operated 844 individual transplant programs. (See table 1.) Nearly all states had at least one transplant center, but some types of transplant programs, such as lung or intestine transplant programs, were located in a limited number of states.

Table 1. Number of Organ Transplant Centers and Programs, 2008

Total number of organ transplant centers	254
Number of organ transplant centers with	
Kidney programs	245
Liver programs	126
Pancreas programsa	175
Heart programs	132
Lung programs	66
Heart-lung programs	54
Intestine programs	46
Total number of organ transplant programs	844

Source: The OPTN.

Notes: Data are as of January 23, 2008. Data on transplant centers that perform heart-lung transplants are captured in a separate category. Data on transplant centers that perform multi-organ transplants other than heart-lung transplants are captured under both organs involved.

[a] Pancreas programs include programs performing transplants of pancreas islet cells.

Organ Transplantation Process

The organ transplantation process involves the following steps.

Step 1: The process begins when a patient's physician determines that an organ transplant may be necessary and refers the patient to a transplant program for evaluation.

Step 2: If the transplant program determines that the patient is a candidate for transplantation, the individual is registered on the national organ transplant waiting list maintained by the OPTN.

Step 3: When an organ becomes available, the local organ procurement organization enters information about the donor organ into a national computer system operated by the OPTN. The computer system generates a ranked list of potential recipients based on how closely their medical characteristics—such as blood type, organ size, and genetic makeup—match the donor's, as well as on the urgency of their medical conditions, their time spent on the waiting list, and their proximity to the donor.[11]

Step 4: Transplant programs whose patients appear on the list are contacted. The decision whether to accept an organ rests with the patient's transplant team. Because the length of time organs can viably be kept outside the body is limited, the transplant team has 1 hour to make its decision. If the organ is not accepted, it is offered to the center with the next patient on the list until the organ is placed.

Step 5: Once the organ is accepted for a potential recipient, a surgical team comes to the donor hospital to recover the organ. The recovered organ is transported from the donor to the recipient hospital for transplantation into the patient.

The OPTN's Role and Responsibilities

The OPTN was created pursuant to the National Organ Transplant Act, which called for HHS to provide by contract for the establishment and operation of the OPTN to manage the nation's organ allocation system.[12] Prior to that time, national policies regarding transplantation did not exist and organ allocation was carried out on an ad hoc basis. The OPTN's functions include maintaining a list of patients waiting for transplants, operating a system for matching donated organs with individuals on the list, establishing medical criteria for allocating organs, collecting and analyzing data on organs donated and transplanted, and conducting work to increase the supply of donated organs. The OPTN's members include all transplant centers and organ procurement organizations in the country; tissue-typing laboratories;[13] professional scientific and medical organizations; and other organizations and individuals interested in organ donation or transplantation, such as organ donors, recipients, and their families. The OPTN's Membership and Professional Standards Committee (MPSC) is responsible for overseeing the compliance of OPTN members with applicable federal regulations and OPTN policies. The OPTN collects most of the funding to cover its operating costs (estimated to be about $25 million in 2006) from candidate registration fees paid by OPTN members; HRSA's funding for the OPTN is capped at $2 million a year.[14]

From early in its history, the OPTN has been responsible for operating an equitable nationwide system of organ allocation. The OPTN develops detailed policies that govern the distribution of organs and other issues related to transplantation, such as the specific credentials required of transplant surgeons and physicians. HHS clarified the OPTN's oversight responsibilities in regulations implemented in 2000.[15] The regulations require the OPTN to design plans and procedures for conducting ongoing and periodic reviews of all member transplant centers for compliance with the regulations and OPTN policies. The regulations also require the OPTN to advise the Secretary of Health and Human Services when the results of its reviews indicate noncompliance with the regulations or OPTN policies or otherwise indicate a risk to patient health or public safety.

While the OPTN is required to monitor transplant programs' compliance with its policies, OPTN policies are considered voluntary or advisory.[16] To promote transplant programs' voluntary compliance with OPTN policies, the OPTN employs a confidential review process in which OPTN members evaluate the medical care provided by colleagues to determine compliance with OPTN policies and regulations.[17] The OPTN emphasizes that its confidential review process focuses on corrective action rather than punishment and is aimed at continuous quality and performance improvement. On its own, the OPTN can impose certain sanctions against noncompliant transplant programs, such as issuing a letter of warning or placing a program on probation. The OPTN can also request that the Secretary of Health and Human Services impose stronger enforcement actions, including terminating a program's ability to receive organs or reimbursement under Medicare.

HRSA's Oversight of the OPTN

The OPTN contract with HRSA includes several requirements related to the oversight of transplant programs. For example, the contract requires the OPTN to conduct on-site reviews of heart, liver, and lung transplant programs at least once every 3 years and to perform ongoing analyses of organ allocations.[18] The OPTN is also required to submit monthly reports to HRSA describing transplant program-specific instances of noncompliance with OPTN policies and the status of corrective action plans. To ensure that the OPTN is fulfilling its responsibilities to monitor transplant programs' compliance, HRSA officials participate as ex officio nonvoting members on the OPTN's Board of Directors and committees, including the MPSC. According to HRSA officials, the agency's presence on OPTN committees helps ensure that the committees' recommendations are consistent with federal laws and regulations. In addition, HRSA officials said that they and OPTN officials communicate regularly about all aspects of the OPTN's performance, including monitoring transplant program compliance.

CMS's Role and Responsibilities

CMS is responsible for overseeing organ transplant programs that receive Medicare reimbursement for transplant services. At the time the high- profile cases came to light, CMS had different criteria and procedures for overseeing extra-renal and renal transplant programs participating in Medicare.

- Extra-renal transplant programs participated in Medicare by meeting the criteria set forth in various national coverage determinations (NCD) published beginning in 1987.[19] The NCDs provide that transplants of extra- renal organs for Medicare beneficiaries will be considered reasonable and necessary and therefore reimbursable under Medicare if they are performed in a facility that CMS approves as meeting specified criteria. For example, heart, liver, and lung transplant programs were required to have written patient selection criteria, perform a minimum number of transplants each year, and meet minimum patient survival rates. The NCDs for these programs did not include criteria for reevaluating the ongoing performance of Medicare-approved programs.
- Renal transplant programs participated in Medicare by meeting regulatory standards for facilities furnishing end-stage renal disease (ESRD) services.[20] ESRD facilities include those providing dialysis services and renal transplant services.[21] CMS monitored renal transplant programs' compliance with Medicare requirements by contracting with state survey agencies—generally state departments of health—to conduct routine on- site inspections known as surveys.[22] If a survey found a facility to be out of compliance and if it had a major deficiency that went uncorrected, then the facility was subject to termination from the Medicare program.

In 2005, recognizing the need to update existing requirements for extra- renal and renal transplant programs and that the NCDs did not include criteria for reassessing the performance of extra-renal transplant programs, CMS promulgated proposed regulations to establish a single set of Medicare requirements for both renal and extra-renal transplant programs.[23]

Limitations Existed in Federal Oversight at the Time High-Profile Problems Came to Light

CMS's and, to a lesser extent, the OPTN's oversight of transplant programs was not comprehensive at the time high-profile problems came to light in 2005 and 2006. CMS did not actively monitor extra-renal transplant programs' compliance with criteria for Medicare approval. CMS monitored renal transplant programs through contracts with state agencies, but the surveys reviewed compliance with requirements that had not been substantially updated in decades and were limited in scope; also, not all programs were actively monitored. At the same time, the OPTN actively monitored transplant programs and took action to resolve identified problems, but its oversight activities fell short in some respects—the OPTN's monitoring did not include methods capable of promptly detecting problems at transplant programs that prolonged the time that patients waited for transplants, and the OPTN did not always meet its goals for conducting on-site reviews.

CMS's Oversight Was Limited and Inconsistent

CMS's oversight varied between extra-renal and renal transplant programs and was not comprehensive even for renal transplant programs, which received more oversight.

CMS Did Not Actively Monitor Extra-Renal Transplant Programs

At the time high-profile problems came to light in 2005 and 2006, CMS was not actively monitoring the ongoing compliance of Medicare-approved extra-renal transplant programs with the criteria specified in the NCDs, which included performing a minimum number of transplants per year and achieving a minimum patient survival rate.[24] Instead, CMS's procedure was to conduct only an initial review of an extra-renal program to determine if it met the criteria in the NCDs at the time the program applied for Medicare approval. Once an extra-renal transplant program received Medicare approval, CMS generally did not assess the program's continued compliance with NCD criteria.[25] Although the NCDs for heart and liver transplant programs called for programs to submit an application for Medicare reapproval every 3 years, the NCDs did not specify and CMS did not otherwise establish a process for doing so, and programs continued to retain Medicare approval without reapplying.

To oversee extra-renal transplant programs' ongoing compliance with criteria for Medicare approval, CMS relied on programs to self-report significant changes and complaints from Medicare beneficiaries and others that would alert CMS to a potential problem. CMS officials or state surveyors conducted complaint investigations after receiving complaints against transplant programs or otherwise becoming aware of potential problems, such as through media reports. CMS officials in three of the five regions we contacted reported that they or state surveyors had investigated nine complaints against extra-renal transplant programs during the period of 2000 through 2006.[26] For example, one of the three high-profile cases initially came to light after CMS received a patient complaint about a liver transplant program. CMS officials investigated the complaint and discovered that this transplant program had not had a full- time surgeon on staff in over a year. After completing the complaint investigation, CMS withdrew Medicare approval from the transplant program, which closed shortly thereafter.

CMS Had a Process in Place to Monitor Renal Transplant Programs, but Some Programs Still Were Not Actively Reviewed

CMS's oversight of renal transplant programs was more active than its oversight of extra-renal transplant programs, although it also had limitations. CMS contracted with state agencies to periodically perform on-site surveys of renal transplant programs for compliance with Medicare requirements and had a process in place to resolve problems identified during these surveys. When state surveyors identified compliance problems with requirements during their reviews of renal transplant programs, CMS generally acted to resolve these problems by requiring programs to submit corrective action plans for coming back into compliance with requirements. According to CMS data, major problems were generally corrected within 90 days, and only one of the five CMS regional offices we contacted reported that CMS had withdrawn Medicare approval from a renal transplant program in its region since 2000 for failure to comply with Medicare requirements. This instance was the high-profile case involving an HMO that was unable to properly handle a large influx of patients to its program.

Although CMS had a process in place to periodically review renal transplant programs through state agency surveys of ESRD facilities, the surveys reviewed compliance with requirements that had not been substantially updated in decades and were limited in scope. Medicare regulations for ESRD facilities, including renal transplant programs, were initially published in 1976 and, according to CMS officials, had not been substantially updated since then.[27] For example, the regulations did not include a requirement that renal transplant programs achieve a minimum patient survival rate. Experts in the transplantation field have since recognized the importance of patient-centered, outcome-oriented performance measures, such as survival rates, and recommended their use.[28] In addition, while the Medicare requirements specified that renal transplant programs should perform a minimum number of transplants per year, CMS instructions to state surveyors did not call for them to verify that these numbers were achieved.[29]

Furthermore, CMS's process to review renal transplant programs did not ensure that all of these programs were actively monitored in practice. Our analysis of CMS data as of

May 2007 showed that 31, or about 1 in 8, active, Medicare-approved renal transplant programs had been mistakenly classified as no longer participating in Medicare in CMS's survey database or had been mistakenly excluded from the database.[30] According to CMS officials, these programs would not have been surveyed again after these mistakes occurred. Our analysis showed that as of May 2007 the length of time since the 31 programs had last been surveyed ranged from about 4 to over 20 years; over three-quarters of these programs had not been surveyed in the previous 10 years. By comparison, most correctly classified programs had been surveyed in the previous 4 years, although 34 programs had not, and 9 of those programs had not been surveyed in the previous 10 years. CMS did not have survey frequency goals specific to renal transplant programs. However, CMS has acknowledged that not all state agencies achieved CMS goals for conducting surveys of all ESRD facilities (of which renal transplant programs are a subset).[31] CMS officials emphasized that the CMS survey and certification budget had not been fully funded during fiscal years 2005 through 2007.

The OPTN's Oversight Was Active and Multipronged but Was Not Sufficient to Detect All Problems

The OPTN's oversight, while more active and extensive than CMS's oversight, also had limitations; most notably, its monitoring methods were insufficient to promptly detect problems affecting patients waiting for transplants.

The OPTN Actively Monitored for Many Types of Problems

The OPTN monitored transplant programs on an ongoing basis for numerous types of potential problems. The OPTN's oversight was conducted by both OPTN staff and by its MPSC, which includes OPTN members who are medical professionals from the field of transplantation. The OPTN's numerous activities to monitor compliance with OPTN policies included reviewing information on patients placed on transplant waiting lists, allocations of organs from deceased donors, physician credentials, and timely submission of required data. These reviews were generally scheduled to occur weekly or quarterly. The OPTN also monitored on a quarterly basis two key indicators of potential performance problems at transplant programs—lower-than-expected patient and organ survival rates and failure to perform any transplants during a specified period of time. In addition, the OPTN conducted periodic routine on-site reviews of heart and liver transplant programs to review patient medical records; the OPTN's goal was to conduct these on- site reviews once every 3 years.[32]

The OPTN's monitoring activities identified many problems, ranging from minor anomalies with organ allocations to more significant problems, including one of the three high-profile cases. The case came to light after a routine OPTN on-site review led staff at the transplant program to self- report that a recipient of a liver transplant had inappropriately received the transplant ahead of others on the waiting list and that the program had falsified patient medical records in order to conceal its actions.[33] Our review of a sample of compliance cases showed that the OPTN most often identified members' noncompliance with OPTN policies through its routine on-site reviews (15 of 43 cases).

Our review of OPTN compliance cases and performance data and discussions with OPTN officials indicated that the OPTN took steps to resolve compliance and performance problems it identified during its monitoring activities. As explained below, the OPTN's process for resolving members' noncompliance with OPTN policies differs from its process for resolving members' performance problems, such as lower-than-expected survival rates.

- *Noncompliance with OPTN policies.* OPTN officials emphasize that the OPTN works to resolve most cases of noncompliance without resorting to strong enforcement actions. Our review of a sample of compliance cases showed that the length of time for cases to be fully resolved varied and depended on the nature of the case. For example, a relatively minor case involving an organ allocation discrepancy was resolved within 4 months, while a case involving problems with medical record documentation took about 3 years to resolve. The three high-profile cases are examples of cases in which the OPTN took strong enforcement actions. After the individual transplant programs involved in these cases had announced that they would voluntarily close, the OPTN continued to review the cases and eventually declared two of the transplant centers that operated these transplant programs "Members Not in Good Standing" and imposed a lesser sanction of probation on the third transplant center.
- *Performance problems.* The OPTN flags for the MPSC's review transplant programs that are not achieving OPTN performance standards for survival rates or transplant activity, but these programs are not considered to be out of compliance with OPTN policies. Instead, the OPTN works with these programs until they meet the standards, sometimes sending peer review teams on-site to consult with the programs, or until problems are otherwise resolved (for example, if a program closes voluntarily). OPTN officials said that

programs with low survival rates typically need to show improvement in outcomes before being released from review by the MPSC and emphasized that this can take some time. Of 72 cases the OPTN flagged for low survival rates in 2005, about 40 percent remained under review by the MPSC as of August 2007.

The OPTN's Monitoring Did Not Detect All High-Profile Cases and Was Not Always Timely

Although the OPTN conducted numerous types of monitoring activities, these activities did not incorporate methods capable of promptly detecting problems at transplant programs that prolonged the time that patients waited for transplants. For example, the OPTN regularly flagged programs for review that did not perform any transplants in a specified period of time.[34] While helpful in detecting completely inactive programs, this particular method did not identify more subtle problems, such as a transplant program that was understaffed and was turning down organs offered for patients at markedly high rates. At the two transplant programs with high-profile problems affecting patient access to transplants, enough transplants were conducted that the programs were not flagged as inactive programs. In addition, the transplants that did occur were successful enough that the programs were not flagged as experiencing performance problems at the time the problems came to light.[35] However, far fewer transplants were conducted than would be expected given the numbers of patients on the waiting list, reflecting problems with understaffing that ultimately affected patients' access to transplants at these programs.

Even though a targeted method for detecting these problems was not in place, separate pieces of information, if pieced together, could have alerted the OPTN to at least one of the high-profile incidents. The OPTN, however, missed opportunities to link these separate sources of information. For example, OPTN staff who handle patient transfers were aware that an HMO was attempting to transfer hundreds of patients to its new transplant program at an unprecedented rate and was experiencing problems with the transfers. However, they did not alert other appropriate OPTN staff to the possible need for a compliance review or to look into the situation by, for example, reviewing available data that indicated far lower-than-expected numbers of transplants at the new program. The problem eventually came to light after a whistleblower alerted the news media.

In addition to having insufficient methods to detect some of the high- profile cases, the OPTN was not always timely in conducting those monitoring activities that it performs on-site, namely routine on-site reviews and peer review site visits. Although the OPTN's goal was to conduct routine on-site reviews of heart and liver programs once every 3 years, it had fallen behind this schedule. In December 2006, 50 percent of continuously active heart and liver transplant programs had not been reviewed on-site in the previous 3 years and 38 percent had not been reviewed on-site in the previous 4 years. OPTN and HRSA officials attribute the delay in routine on-site reviews to HRSA's directive to the OPTN to study a new lung allocation policy. Additionally, in our review of performance data we observed that in some cases peer review site visits were not conducted on a timely basis. For about three-fourths of transplant programs (17 of 22) for which the MPSC recommended a peer review site visit from July 2005 through July 2006, the site visit had not yet occurred a year after being recommended. According to OPTN officials, a contributing factor in the delay was that the number of programs recommended to receive a peer review site visit significantly increased during 2005, resulting in a backlog.[36]

CMS, HRSA, AND THE OPTN HAVE ACTED TO STRENGTHEN OVERSIGHT, BUT THE FULL EFFECT OF THESE ACTIONS WILL DEPEND ON IMPLEMENTATION AND FURTHER INFORMATION SHARING

Since the high-profile cases came to light, CMS, HRSA, and the OPTN have made some changes and planned others to improve federal oversight of organ transplant programs; however, the full effect of these changes remains to be seen. CMS has begun monitoring extra-renal transplant programs and has finalized regulations that expand and unify Medicare requirements for all types of transplant programs and establish procedures for periodic review of transplant programs. The OPTN and HRSA are working to develop and implement a set of indicators to help the OPTN better identify problems that prolong the time patients wait for transplants. Implementation of CMS's new requirements is in its early stages, however, and CMS has not resolved the extent to which on-site surveys will be performed as part of its periodic reviews of programs for Medicare reapproval. Also, the OPTN's and HRSA's set of indicators has not yet been implemented. Further, while CMS, HRSA, and the OPTN have begun sharing basic transplant program data, how they will share additional information resulting from their oversight activities has not been resolved.

CMS Strengthened Oversight by Expanding Monitoring Efforts and Issuing New Regulations

CMS has made substantial changes to its oversight: the agency began monitoring extra-renal transplant programs and, most significantly, finalized new regulations that apply to all types of transplant programs and that require on-site surveys of all transplant programs applying for Medicare approval.

CMS Began Monitoring Extra- Renal Transplant Programs and Took Steps to Withdraw Medicare Approval from the Most Problematic Programs

After high-profile problems came to light, CMS began monitoring extra- renal transplant programs' compliance with existing Medicare NCD criteria in 2006. According to CMS officials, the agency's initial monitoring effort revealed that nearly all 242 Medicare-approved programs were complying with NCD criteria for meeting minimum survival rates. A number of programs, however, were not in compliance with the NCD annual transplant volume criteria, which specify that programs must conduct a minimum number of transplants each year. CMS continued to monitor extra-renal transplant programs and ultimately found that a total of 49 extra-renal transplant programs did not meet the NCD transplant volume criteria in 2005, 2006, or both. As a result, CMS notified 11 programs that agency officials viewed as the most problematic that they could lose Medicare approval for failure to comply with NCD criteria.[37] Ultimately, CMS withdrew Medicare approval from 1 of the 11 programs; of the remaining 10 programs, 2 withdrew voluntarily and 8 programs were implementing corrective action plans as of December 2007. (See table 2.)

Table 2. Status of the 49 Extra-Renal Transplant Programs That Did Not Meet NCD Volume Criteria in 2005, 2006, or Both

11	Noncompliant programs were notified by CMS that they could lose Medicare approval for failure to comply with NCD criteria
2	Programs voluntarily withdrew from Medicare
8	Programs submitted corrective action plans that were approved by CMS
1	Program submitted a corrective action plan that CMS rejected (Medicare approval was withdrawn)
38	Noncompliant programs were not notified by CMS
5	Programs voluntarily withdrew from Medicare
12	Programs improved and met transplant volume criteria in 2006
11	Programs met or were projected to meet transplant volume criteria in 2007
10	Programs were projected to remain out of compliance with volume criteria in 2007

Source: GAO analysis of information provided by CMS.

CMS Established New Requirements that Apply to All Types of Transplant Programs

In March 2007, CMS made a more fundamental change to its oversight by publishing final regulations establishing a new set of Medicare requirements specifically for organ transplant programs. The regulations include 13 core requirements known as Medicare conditions of participation (CoP). Whereas renal and extra-renal transplant programs were previously subject to different requirements and regulatory procedures, the new regulations provide a single set of CoPs and review procedures for all types of transplant programs. In addition, the new regulations both update and expand upon previous requirements. For example, the new CoPs incorporate an updated method for calculating survival rates that reflects current best practices. The CoPs also include entirely new requirements, such as those related to the protection of living donors. (See app. I for more information about the 13 CoPs.)

The new regulations also bring CMS requirements into substantial alignment with OPTN policies. Specifically, 10 of the 13 CoPs pertain to areas addressed in OPTN policies. In some instances, CMS incorporated OPTN policies into its requirements such that these policies are now enforceable under federal regulation for Medicare-approved transplant programs. In some areas, the new regulations impose additional requirements not covered by the OPTN. For example, while OPTN policies require transplant programs to provide social support services, CMS's regulations further require that social support services be furnished by a qualified social worker, as defined by CMS. In other areas, the new CMS requirements cover matters not addressed in existing OPTN policies. For example, one CoP requires programs to implement formal quality assessment and performance improvement programs—a requirement not paralleled in OPTN policies. There are also areas of OPTN policies, largely pertaining to organ allocation, which the CMS regulations do not address.

New Regulations Also Established Procedures for Reviewing Transplant Programs

In addition to updating and expanding requirements and more closely aligning them with OPTN policies, CMS's new regulations also subject transplant programs to initial and periodic reviews for compliance with the Medicare CoPs. Under the new regulations, all transplant programs seeking Medicare approval are required to apply for initial approval; programs that were previously Medicare approved must reapply.[38] As part of determining compliance with the CoPs, each transplant program that applies for Medicare approval will undergo an on-site survey. Transplant programs that are in compliance with all CoPs will be approved for participation in Medicare for 3 years. Prior to the end of the initial 3-year approval period,

CMS plans to reexamine data on three key requirements, which together compose one of the CoPs:[39]

- Data submission: Transplant programs must submit OPTN-required data to the OPTN within specified time frames.
- Clinical experience: Transplant programs must generally perform at least 10 transplants over a 12-month period.
- Outcomes: Transplant programs must achieve expected survival rates.[40]

If a program is found to be in compliance with the three requirements of this CoP, under the new regulations CMS may choose whether to conduct an on-site reapproval survey of the program's compliance with additional CoPs.

CMS plans to complete on-site surveys for transplant programs seeking initial Medicare approval over the course of 3 years. CMS officials reported that on-site surveys of transplant programs had begun as of August 2007. The agency is prioritizing the order in which these surveys will be conducted, so that programs that do not currently meet the clinical experience and outcomes requirements will receive the highest priority for surveys.[41] According to CMS officials, the agency plans to complete these high-priority surveys by the end of fiscal year 2008; all initial surveys are planned to be completed by the end of fiscal year 2010. Until a new Medicare approval decision is made under the new regulations, currently approved extra-renal and renal transplant programs will remain approved under the NCDs and requirements for ESRD facilities, respectively.[42]

The OPTN and HRSA Have Taken Steps to Address Shortcomings in Detection of Problems

To address shortcomings in the OPTN's ability to detect problems affecting patients waiting for transplants, such as understaffing, the OPTN and HRSA, along with another HRSA contractor, are working to develop and implement a set of activity-level indicators. The set of indicators would be used to monitor programs for problems, such as understaffing, indicated by lower-than-expected activity levels in a manner similar to how the OPTN currently monitors programs for performance problems indicated by lower-than-expected survival rates. The set of indicators includes two existing indicators already developed by the OPTN, one of which, although available, was not previously reviewed by the MPSC, and a new organ acceptance rate indicator. The new indicator, which is intended to identify programs exhibiting lower-than-expected rates of organ acceptance, is a key component of the set of activity-level indicators and has been under development since January 2006. According to the OPTN, the organ acceptance rate indicator had been developed but not yet implemented for kidney and liver transplant programs as of February 2008.

With HRSA's encouragement, the OPTN has also taken steps to increase its capacity to conduct on-site monitoring activities and to improve internal communication. The OPTN substantially increased its staff in 2007 in order to get back on schedule in conducting on-site reviews once every 3 years. According to OPTN officials, the increase in staff will also help the OPTN address its backlog of peer review site visits and achieve its goal of conducting all peer review site visits within 3 months of the visit being recommended by the MPSC. To improve internal communication, the OPTN reported that since 2006, its leadership has emphasized the importance of shared communication, particularly across departments. As a result, according to the OPTN, staff responsible for managing the waiting list, including handling patient transfers, now meet frequently with staff responsible for monitoring policy compliance to share information about potential policy violations.

CMS, HRSA, and the OPTN Have Yet to Fully Implement Several Measures to Improve Oversight

Although CMS, HRSA, and the OPTN have taken steps to improve oversight of transplant programs since the high-profile cases came to light, three important areas remain in progress.

- One key unresolved question is the extent to which CMS will conduct on-site reapproval surveys of transplant programs (as part of its new review procedures) after transplant programs gain initial Medicare approval under the new regulations. According to CMS's new regulations, CMS may choose not to conduct on-site reapproval surveys for transplant programs meeting data submission, clinical experience, and outcomes requirements. This means that CMS could potentially choose not to conduct any reapproval surveys for programs meeting these requirements. While CMS officials said that they see value in conducting reapproval surveys, just how CMS will apply its discretion remains unclear. As of January 2008, CMS officials said that the agency had not decided how many reapproval surveys it would conduct or how it would choose which programs to survey among those that meet the aforementioned requirements. They emphasized the agency's need to carefully consider resource constraints in making these decisions. A decision by CMS not to conduct an on-site reapproval survey at a transplant program means that compliance with some CoPs would not be reviewed unless there was a complaint investigation. As a result, problems at transplant programs unrelated to the data submission, clinical experience, and outcomes requirements—for example, a transplant program failing to provide required protections for living donors or to sufficiently staff its program—could go undetected. In two of the high-profile cases, staffing problems that ultimately affected patients' access to transplants would not have been detected by the outcomes indicator that CMS has now adopted, and the numbers of transplants performed per year at these programs exceeded or were close to CMS's clinical experience requirement.

- Additional questions remain regarding the extent to which CMS will accurately track on-site surveys to avoid the misclassification errors we identified in our review and complete the surveys on a timely basis. As a result of the new transplant regulations, renal transplant programs will no longer share Medicare identification numbers with dialysis facilities, and previously misclassified renal transplant programs will at some point receive a new accurate classification in CMS's survey database once they are approved. However, the potential for transplant programs to be mistakenly classified may remain because transplant programs within the same hospital will share one transplant center Medicare identification number, according to CMS officials. CMS officials said that they were highly aware of the need for their systems to accurately track the status of each transplant program separately. They said that they plan to test for this capability in their new tracking system for transplant programs, which remains under development. What also remains to be seen is the extent to which surveys will occur on a timely basis. Prior to the new regulations, state agencies did not always meet CMS goals for surveying ESRD facilities. Now, under the new regulations, the responsibilities of state agencies that will be conducting on-site surveys of transplant programs will increase, since they will be required to survey both renal and extra- renal transplant programs.[43] With respect to initial approval surveys, CMS's stated plan is that high-priority surveys of transplant programs will be completed by the end of fiscal year 2008, but as of January 2008, CMS officials expressed some uncertainty about meeting this goal. Initial surveys of transplant programs have been given a relatively high priority in the state agency workload, but it is not definite that this high priority level will continue because CMS has revised state agency workload priorities in the past.[44] Further, the priority level for reapproval surveys is not yet known; a lower priority could affect how frequently surveys occur.

- The last unresolved question concerns the OPTN's and HRSA's planned organ acceptance rate indicator, which as part of a set of activity-level indicators, could potentially improve the OPTN's ability to detect transplant programs experiencing problems that prolong the time patients wait for transplants. According to the OPTN, the organ acceptance rate indicator for kidney and liver transplant programs has been developed but, as of February 2008, has not yet been implemented; HRSA officials expect the indicator to be in place within 1 year. HRSA and OPTN officials reported that they are considering developing organ acceptance rate indicators for transplant programs for other organ types. Before extending the indicator to other types of programs, however, the OPTN will first assess the effectiveness of the indicator at detecting potential problems at kidney and liver transplant programs, which perform larger volumes of transplants, and determine the feasibility of developing an indicator for programs with lower transplant volumes, such as heart and lung transplant programs.

CMS, HRSA, and the OPTN Are Sharing Basic Data on Transplant Programs, but How They Will Share Additional Information from Their Oversight Activities Has Not Been Resolved

CMS, HRSA, and the OPTN have recognized the importance of sharing data on transplant programs with one another and have taken initial steps to share basic data. To help CMS assess programs' compliance with its new Medicare requirements, the OPTN (through HRSA) is now sending CMS certain basic transplant program data on a quarterly basis.[45] For example, the new Medicare regulations require transplant centers to be OPTN members, so the OPTN is providing data on the status of each transplant center's membership in the OPTN. (See table 3.)

While this basic data sharing represents progress, CMS, HRSA, and the OPTN have additional information resulting from their oversight activities that could be shared. The exchange of this information is important because CMS and the OPTN conduct different monitoring activities and, as a result, may have different information about transplant programs that could be relevant to each other. For example, while both CMS and the OPTN conduct on-site reviews of transplant programs, the OPTN's on-site reviews focus largely on medical records review while CMS's on-site surveys are more broadly scoped. If the OPTN determined during an on-site review that the medical urgency assigned to patients by a transplant program was not supported by its medical records, this information could be of interest to CMS if this practice inappropriately reduced the chances of others on the waiting list to receive a transplant. As another example, the OPTN and HRSA are working to put into place their organ acceptance rate indicator, which CMS officials said they would be interested in using. Information from CMS's and the OPTN's investigations could also be potentially important to share. For example, if CMS investigated a complaint from a patient about the length of time he or she had been waiting for a transplant and determined that the delay was caused by the program failing to update the patient's health status, a violation of OPTN policy, the OPTN might want to flag the program for closer monitoring.

Table 3. Medicare Requirements for Transplant Programs for Which the OPTN Is Providing Data to CMS

Medicare requirement	Data provided to CMS on each OPTN member
Transplant programs must be a member of the OPTN	OPTN membership status
Transplant programs must submit OPTN-required data to the OPTN within 90 days of OPTN deadlines	Member's compliance with OPTN data submission policies
The hospital in which a transplant program operates must have a written agreement with an organ procurement organization to receive organs	The organ procurement organization with which the transplant center has an agreement
Transplant programs must ensure that all individuals who provide services at the program, supervise services, or both are qualified to provide or supervise such services	The names of the primary surgeon and primary physician at the transplant program

Source: GAO analysis of Medicare CoPs for transplant centers and information from CMS and HRSA.

CMS and HRSA have recognized the importance of sharing information from their oversight activities, but the agencies have not yet reached agreement on how they would do so. CMS submitted a draft proposal to HRSA in April 2007 describing how CMS and HRSA could potentially share information about organ transplant programs. CMS and HRSA officials have since discussed the initial proposal, including possible revisions, but their progress has been slow. As of February 2008, CMS and HRSA had yet to reach agreement or establish a time frame for doing so. According to HRSA officials it had taken the agencies several months to better understand each other's oversight processes, and both agencies needed to further explore their information needs. CMS officials also indicated that further issues would need to be resolved before an agreement could be reached.

As part of any agreement to share information from their oversight activities, CMS and HRSA will need to determine precisely what information from their oversight activities they will share and at what point in their oversight processes they will share it. CMS and HRSA have discussed but not resolved these issues:

- *Nature of information to be shared.* It will be important for CMS and HRSA to determine specifically what information they will share from their oversight activities. For example, while CMS's initial proposal addressed how CMS and HRSA could share information from CMS's and the OPTN's investigations of serious complaints, such as those involving threats to patient health and safety, CMS and HRSA officials have since discussed whether to share information from all complaints. In addition, CMS and HRSA have not determined to what extent information from routine inspections, such as the OPTN's on-site reviews and CMS's on-site surveys, will be shared and at what level of detail. For example, CMS's initial proposal called for CMS to notify the OPTN about its completed on- site surveys and to indicate whether the transplant program surveyed had a plan of correction, but it did not call for CMS to provide information on the deficiencies CMS found. HRSA officials have since expressed their interest in having this more detailed information.
- *Timing of information sharing.* A more difficult challenge that CMS and HRSA face is agreeing when to share information about potential problems at transplant programs. Officials from both CMS and HRSA consider the severity of the identified problem(s) with a program to be a key factor in determining the appropriate time for information sharing. In this regard, officials from both agencies stated a willingness to promptly share information on potentially serious problems. Agreeing on just when to exchange information on less serious problems has been more problematic for the agencies in part because of differences in their approaches to oversight. On the one hand, CMS officials emphasize their agency's obligation to investigate any indications of noncompliance with Medicare requirements and prefer to be notified as soon as possible if the OPTN discovers a potential problem indicating noncompliance with Medicare CoPs. On the other hand, HRSA officials have emphasized that the viability and success of the OPTN's performance improvement process depends upon transplant programs sharing openly about their practices or past events. HRSA officials contend that the possibility of such information being shared with CMS, a regulatory agency, could cause transplant programs to be less candid about discussing real or

potential problems, making it more difficult for the OPTN to help them return to compliance.

CONCLUSIONS

CMS, HRSA, and the OPTN recognize the gaps in oversight that existed when serious problems were exposed at transplant centers and have taken significant steps to strengthen federal oversight. The actions they have taken will help improve standards for transplant programs and should improve detection of potential problems. These actions include CMS's issuance of new regulations that expand and update requirements for transplant programs. In addition, CMS plans to conduct on-site surveys of all transplant programs seeking initial Medicare approval under the new regulations and to regularly review certain transplant program data, which should reduce the chances of problems going undetected by the agency. Similarly, if the OPTN's and HRSA's efforts to develop and implement a set of activity-level indicators to detect problems that prolong the time patients wait for transplants are successful, the indicators will likely result in earlier detection of these more subtle problems.

The full effect of these planned improvements, however, is unknown at this time, and much has yet to be accomplished. While surveyors have begun conducting on-site surveys for initial Medicare approval, CMS expects these surveys may take 3 years to complete. CMS is still in the process of designing its tracking system for transplant programs, and it is important that the system include mechanisms to check that transplant programs remain accurately classified in the CMS survey database over time. The OPTN and HRSA are working on implementing their set of activity-level indicators for kidney and liver transplant programs. It will be important for the OPTN and HRSA to implement the activity-level indicators to the extent feasible to provide improved monitoring tools to detect problems affecting patient access to transplants like those involved in the high-profile cases in 2005 and 2006. Attending to these areas is critical for effective oversight, and we encourage CMS, HRSA, and the OPTN to continue their efforts to implement these initiatives.

Of more concern are two other issues. The first is how CMS will ultimately conduct on-site surveys for transplant programs seeking reapproval under the new Medicare regulations. Under the regulations, CMS may choose not to conduct such surveys for transplant programs meeting data submission, clinical experience, and outcomes requirements. Not conducting on-site reapproval surveys may limit CMS's ability to monitor these transplant programs' compliance with other Medicare CoPs, for example, whether transplant programs are providing required protections for living donors, and to detect problems like those involved in some of the high-profile cases. CMS has not yet developed a process to determine the scope of the transplant programs (number or type) to be included in reapproval surveys or the criteria for determining which, if any, transplant programs that meet the three requirements will receive such surveys. Given the potential importance of these reapproval surveys, we believe that having a methodology that ensures that CMS conducts surveys of at least some transplant programs meeting the three requirements is critical to maximize CMS's opportunities to identify potential problems in a timely manner.

We also have a concern about the pace of progress being made to share information about the oversight activities of CMS, HRSA, and the OPTN. Agency officials believe, as we do, that their ability to identify potential problems could be enhanced by sharing information resulting from their oversight activities. While CMS's draft proposal for sharing such information is an important first step in reaching an agreement on this issue, CMS and HRSA have yet to finalize an agreement or establish a time frame for doing so. Without a definitive time frame for reaching agreement, there is increased risk that the negotiation process among these agencies could languish, and they could miss opportunities to detect and remedy problems with transplant programs. Furthermore, in developing an agreement, CMS and HRSA will need to fully articulate what types of information will be shared from their oversight activities and when they will share it. While we agree that there are challenges associated with reaching agreement on this issue, we also believe it is important to settle these issues and finalize a clear written agreement that maximizes information sharing as appropriate and better ensures that all parties are aware of critical information in time to take appropriate action. Once CMS and HRSA reach and implement an agreement, they may wish to periodically assess how effectively it is working for each of them to improve their oversight.

Recommendations for Executive Action

To improve federal oversight of organ transplant programs, we recommend that the Secretary of Health and Human Services:

1. Direct the Administrator of CMS to develop a methodology for conducting on-site surveys of transplant programs seeking Medicare reapproval that ensures that at least some transplant programs meeting data submission, clinical experience, and outcomes requirements receive on-site surveys.

2. Direct the Administrators of CMS and HRSA to establish a time frame for finalizing an agreement for the agencies to share information resulting from

CMS's and the OPTN's oversight activities. The agreement should, at a minimum,

- specify the types of information CMS, HRSA, and the OPTN will share and
- specify at what point in CMS's and the OPTN's oversight processes this information will be exchanged.

AGENCY COMMENTS

We received comments on a draft of this report from HHS. (See app. II.) The department concurred with both of our recommendations and commented that CMS recognizes the need to increase its oversight of organ transplant programs.

HHS agreed with our recommendation that CMS develop a methodology for conducting on-site surveys for Medicare reapproval to ensure that at least some programs meeting certain Medicare criteria are surveyed, noting that CMS has developed an initial framework for doing so but that its implementation will depend on the resources available for survey and certification activities. CMS highlighted several factors the agency may use as part of a methodology to determine survey frequencies for individual transplant programs, including prior survey results, program changes, program indicators, and the time interval since the last survey.

HHS also agreed with our recommendation to establish a time frame for finalizing the agreement between HRSA and CMS to share information from their oversight activities, noting that HRSA and CMS have been working to develop and finalize such an agreement. Specifically, the department commented that CMS has conveyed a proposal to HRSA regarding the criteria and process that CMS would use in sharing information, and that CMS would like the agreement with HRSA to be finalized by June 30, 2008. HHS also noted that even though a formal agreement is not yet in place, CMS and HRSA have on several occasions already shared oversight information about particular programs.

The department also provided technical comments, which we incorporated as appropriate.

As arranged with your office, unless you publicly announce the contents of this report earlier, we plan no further distribution of it until 30 days after its date. At that time, we will send copies of this report to the Secretary of Health and Human Services, the Administrators of CMS and HRSA, and appropriate congressional committees. We will also provide copies to others upon request. In addition, the report is available at no charge on the GAO Web site at http://www.gao.gov.

If you or your staff members have any questions about this report, please contact me at (202) 512-7114 or williamsonr@gao.gov. GAO staff who made major contributions to this report are listed in appendix III.

Sincerely yours,

Randall B. Williamson Director, Health Care

APPENDIX I: MEDICARE CONDITIONS OF PARTICIPATION FOR TRANSPLANT CENTERS

On March 30, 2007, the Centers for Medicare & Medicaid Services (CMS) published a final rule promulgating requirements for Medicare approval and reapproval of transplant centers to perform organ transplants. The regulations, which became effective June 28, 2007, delineate Medicare conditions of participation for heart, heart-lung, intestine, kidney, liver, lung, and pancreas transplant centers.[46] Table 4 presents a summary of the key requirements for each condition of participation.

Table 4. Summary of Medicare Conditions of Participation for Transplant Centers

Title of condition of participation	Summary of requirements
Organ Procurement and Transplantation Network (OPTN) membership	The transplant program must be located in a hospital that is a member of the OPTN and that abides by the approved rules and requirements of the OPTN.
Notification to CMS	The transplant program must notify CMS of any significant changes related to the program or changes that could affect its compliance with the Medicare conditions of participation.
Pediatric transplants	A transplant program seeking to perform pediatric transplants must apply for specific approval to do so.
Data submission, clinical experience, and outcomes requirements for initial approval	For initial Medicare approval: • The transplant program must submit required data to the OPTN within a specified time frame. • Adult heart, liver, lung, and intestine transplant programs must generally perform 10 transplants over a 12-month period; adult kidney transplant programs must perform at least 3 transplants over a 12-month period prior to their request for initial approval. • Heart, liver, lung, and kidney transplant programs must have acceptable patient and graft (transplanted organ) survival rates.a

Table 4. (Continued).

Title of condition of participation	Summary of requirements
Data submission, clinical experience, and outcomes requirements for reapproval	To renew Medicare approval: • The transplant program must submit required data to the OPTN within a specified time frame. • Adult heart, liver, lung, intestine, and kidney transplant programs must perform an average of 10 transplants per year. • Heart, liver, lung, and kidney transplant programs must have acceptable patient and graft survival rates.a
Patient and living donor selection	The transplant program must use written patient selection criteria and, if applicable, written living donor selection criteria. Patient selection criteria must assure a nondiscriminatory distribution of organs. Living donor selection criteria must be consistent with principles of medical ethics.
Organ recovery and receipt	The transplant program must have written protocols, including documentation of vital information, for recovery and receipt of organs from deceased donors and for living donor organ transplantation. The transplanting surgeon is responsible for ensuring the medical suitability of organs for transplantation into the intended recipient.
Patient and living donor management	The transplant program must have written patient and, if applicable, living donor management policies; keep patient waiting lists and medical records up to date; and provide social and nutritional services to patients and donors.
Quality assessment and performance improvement	The transplant program must develop, implement, and maintain a quality assessment and performance improvement program to monitor and evaluate its transplantation services.
Human resources	The transplant program must ensure that staff, including the program director, primary transplant surgeon and physician, clinical transplant coordinator, and living donor advocate are qualified and meet CMS-specified requirements.
Organ procurement	The hospital containing the transplant program must have a written agreement with an organ procurement organization designated by the Secretary of Health and Human Services.
Patient and living donor rights	The transplant program must protect and promote patient and living donor rights through the implementation of informed consent policies, and must notify patients about factors that could affect patient access to transplantation, such as termination of Medicare approval or that the program is served by a single surgeon.

Title of condition of participation	Summary of requirements
Additional requirements for kidney transplant centers	Kidney transplant programs must furnish dialysis services and other care to end-stage renal disease patients.

Source: GAO analysis of Medicare hospital conditions of participation for transplant centers.

[a] CMS will compare data on observed patient deaths and graft failures 1-year post-transplant to the expected number of deaths and graft failures 1-year post-transplant calculated by the Scientific Registry of Transplant Recipients, which uses risk-adjusted statistical models. CMS will consider patient and graft survival rates to be unacceptable if the observed patient or survival rate is lower than expected and all three of the following are true: (1) the one-sided p-value is less than 0.05, (2) the number of observed events (patient deaths or graft failures) minus the number of expected events is greater than 3, and (3) the number of observed events divided by the number of expected events is greater than 1.5.

APPENDIX II: COMMENTS FROM THE DEPARTMENT OF HEALTH AND HUMAN SERVICES

DEPARTMENT OF HEALTH & HUMAN SERVICES

Office of the Assistant Secretary for Legislation

Washington, D.C. 20201

APR 14 2008

Randall Williamson
Acting Director, Health Care
U.S. Government Accountability Office
Washington, DC 20548

Dear Mr. Williamson:

Enclosed are the Department's comments on the U.S. Government Accountability Office's (GAO) report entitled: Organ Transplant Programs: Federal Agencies Have Acted to Improve Oversight but Implementation Issues Remain" (GAO 08-412).

The Department appreciates the opportunity to review and comment on this report before its publication.

Sincerely,

Vincent Ventimiglia
Assistant Secretary for Legislation

DEPARTMENT OF HEALTH & HUMAN SERVICES

Centers for Medicare & Medicaid Services

Administrator
Washington, DC 20201

DATE: APR 1 4 2008

TO: Randall Williamson
Acting Director, Health Care
Government Accountability Office

FROM: Kerry Weems
Acting Administrator

SUBJECT: Government Accountability Office (GAO) Draft Report: "Organ Transplant Programs: Federal Agencies Have Acted to Improve Oversight but Implementation Issues Remain" (GAO-08-412)

Thank you for the opportunity to comment on the subject GAO Draft Report. The purpose of the report was to examine--(1) Federal oversight of transplant programs at the time several high-profile organ transplant cases came to light in 2005 and 2006; and (2) changes that Federal agencies have made or planned since then to strengthen oversight.

The Centers for Medicare and Medicaid Services (CMS) recognizes the need to increase our oversight of organ transplant programs, and appreciates GAO's description of our considerable efforts over the past 18 months to strengthen oversight of hospital transplant programs, such as the following:

- ***Review of Extra-Renal Programs under the National Coverage Determinations:*** In 2006, CMS notified 11 extra-renal transplant programs that their Medicare approval was in jeopardy due to failure to comply with the National Coverage Determinations. As discussed in the GAO report, Medicare participation ended (either voluntarily or involuntarily) for 3 of those programs. The remaining 8 programs have submitted corrective action plans that were approved, and continue to be monitored, by CMS.

- ***Release of Regulation Establishing Organ Transplant Conditions of Participation:*** In March 2007, CMS published new Conditions of Participation (CoPs) for organ transplant programs. The CoPs established one set of 13 minimum requirements that all transplant programs must meet in order to participate in Medicare.

- ***Development of Surveyor Guidance:*** In 2007, CMS developed detailed guidance for surveyors who conduct the onsite review of transplant programs to assist in their determination of program compliance with the CoP. This guidance outlines the sources of evidence (e.g., policies, procedures, medical records) that surveyors will review to evaluate compliance with each Condition of the regulation.

- ***Coordination between CMS and the Health Resources and Services Administration (HRSA):*** In April 2007, CMS and HRSA began a dialogue to address the areas where our separate regulatory responsibilities intersect and discuss how coordination/collaboration

Page 2 - Randall Williamson

could reinforce each agency's oversight efforts in this area. CMS and HRSA have agreed to exchange program information quarterly, and are continuing discussions about the exchange of case-specific information (e.g., complaints).

- ***Survey Implementation:*** In August 2007, CMS trained 66 surveyors to perform transplant program surveys. The onsite transplant surveys began in August 2007, and are ongoing. State survey agencies are conducting the surveys in most States, while a national contractor is conducting surveys in others.

- ***Continued Improvement:*** We continue to benefit from feedback from surveyors, professional associations, States, transplant programs, and the public as we review early survey experience and work to improve our interpretive guidance for surveyors.

The GAO report makes two recommendations for the CMS consideration. These recommendations and our responses to these recommendations are listed below.

Recommendation #1: CMS should develop a methodology for conducting on-site surveys for Medicare re-approval to ensure that at least some programs meeting certain Medicare criteria are surveyed.

CMS Response: The CMS concurs with this recommendation. We have already developed an initial framework for doing so, but implementation of the methodology will depend on the resources available for survey and certification (S&C) activities. As you may know, the current level of survey activity for transplant programs was initiated by CMS without explicit fiscal support from Congress. We sincerely hope that the necessary resources will be available to enable us to maintain this level of S&C frequency for transplant programs.

At the present time we are implementing onsite surveys based on a 3-year survey and certification cycle. This means that re-approval surveys will begin in fiscal year (FY) 2010 for those transplant programs first surveyed in FY 2007. Ideally, we would be able to continue the re-certification surveys on the same 3-year cycle, on average, depending on the budget.

However, as discussed in the GAO report, the regulation permits CMS to make future survey and compliance determinations based on other factors. Even with a 3-year survey cycle on average, we plan to adjust survey frequencies for any specific transplant program taking into account past compliance with regulatory requirements. For example, such factors may include the following:

- ***Prior Survey Results:*** In some cases, the findings from a prior survey would warrant more frequent or less frequent onsite review to verify that compliance with the CoP is maintained.

- ***Program Changes***: On an ongoing basis, transplant programs are required to report significant program changes that may affect compliance with the CoP (e.g., key personnel changes, inactivity). Such reports may indicate a period of transition for a transplant program. CMS would want to consider reviewing transplant programs that have been through a significant transition since their last onsite survey to ensure that the CoP continue to be met.

Page 3 - Randall Williamson

- ***Program Indicators:*** Every 6 months, the Scientific Registry of Transplant Recipients (SRTR) publishes reports that provide key program information, such as: outcome data, how long individuals at that program wait for an organ transplant, how many individuals have received transplants, what the patient mortality rate at that program is for individuals on the waiting list, etc. These reports compare a program's information with others in their region and with the national average. We expect that these data would be used to develop indicators where potential issues may exist, and where an onsite review would be most important.

- ***Interval Since the Last Survey:*** After the first re-approval period, CMS will consider the time that has elapsed since a program's last onsite survey, as well as intervening complaints that have been substantiated through a complaint investigation.

Recommendation #2: Establish a timeframe for finalizing the agreement between HRSA and CMS to share information from our oversight activities.

CMS Response: The CMS agrees with this recommendation. CMS and HRSA have been working to develop and finalize an agreement regarding the sharing of information from our mutual oversight activities. We have made significant progress on the content and format for sharing transplant program data on a quarterly basis (as described in the GAO report), and we are hopeful that we are close to an agreement outlining the criteria and process for sharing case-specific notifications of program changes, complaints, and inactivity.

We have conveyed to HRSA a proposal regarding the criteria and process that CMS would use in sharing information regarding specific cases. This would include communicating at an early stage in cases of high-profile incidences, incidences of gross negligence, or a program's inactivity, and routinely sharing CMS survey findings that identify that a program is out of compliance with one or more Medicare CoP. The results of any other survey finding would be shared with HRSA upon request. We hope that the agreement can be finalized between CMS and HRSA by June 30, 2008.

Even though a formal agreement is not yet in place, neither CMS nor HRSA is waiting for such an agreement to work together in sharing information that results from our oversight activities. Since the onsite surveys have started, there have been several occasions where CMS and HRSA have discussed a particular program's status or investigated a complaint that has been referred to us.

We thank the GAO staff for their work in this important area of federal health care purchasing and oversight.

REFERENCES

[1] In 2007, 14,393 individuals (deceased and living) donated one or more organs.

[2] The United Network for Organ Sharing (UNOS), a nonprofit organization, administers the OPTN under contract with HRSA. We use the OPTN to refer to

the OPTN, UNOS, or both and OPTN officials to refer to OPTN officials, UNOS officials responsible for administering the OPTN, or both.

[3] The OPTN's expectations for its members are specified in OPTN policies and OPTN bylaws. In this report, we refer to both OPTN policies and OPTN bylaws as OPTN policies.

[4] CMS was known as the Health Care Financing Administration prior to June 14, 2001. In this report, we use CMS to refer to activities of both CMS and the Heath Care Financing Administration.

[5] Medicare is a federal program that finances health care for people aged 65 years or older and for younger people with disabilities and people with end-stage renal disease (permanent kidney failure requiring dialysis or transplantation).

[6] Based on CMS and OPTN data, we estimate that about 80 percent of transplant programs are Medicare approved.

[7] For purposes of this report, we consider federal agencies' oversight of organ transplant programs to include the oversight activities conducted by CMS, HRSA, and the OPTN.

[8] We excluded from our review oversight of transplant programs under CMS's Medicaid program, the joint federal-state program that finances health care for certain low-income individuals. According to CMS officials, oversight of transplant programs that receive Medicaid reimbursement is handled by state Medicaid programs. We also did not examine the OPTN's, HRSA's, or CMS's oversight of organ procurement organizations, which are responsible for the retrieval, preservation, and transportation of donated organs.

[9] A total of 81 transplant centers had compliance cases from 2003 through 2006. We randomly selected 27 of the 81 centers and supplemented the random sample by including all additional compliance cases from transplant centers where the OPTN took strong enforcement actions from 2000 through 2006 that were not already included in the random sample (4 centers). Some transplant centers had multiple cases reviewed by the OPTN at that time; we reviewed all 43 cases associated with the 31 transplant centers we selected.

[10] Pancreas transplant programs are extra-renal transplant programs, but CMS officials stated that its surveys of renal (kidney) transplant programs are in effect reviews of pancreas transplant programs, noting that Medicare-approved pancreas transplants have largely been performed by Medicare-approved kidney transplant programs. For example, according to CMS, since 2003, no Medicare-approved pancreas transplant had been performed outside of a Medicare-approved kidney transplant program. For the

purposes of this report, when we refer to CMS's monitoring of extra-renal transplant programs we mean its monitoring of heart, liver, lung, and intestine transplant programs.

[11] Medical urgency is measured differently for different organs, according to criteria established by the OPTN, and may include such factors as life expectancy and intensity of current treatment.

[12] Pub. L. No. 98-507, § 201, 98 Stat. 2339, 2342 (1984) (codified as amended at 42 U.S.C. § 274). The Secretary of Health and Human Services delegated this responsibility to HRSA.

[13] Tissue-typing laboratories test potential donors and recipients for tissue compatibility. Tissue typing is routinely performed for all donors and recipients in kidney and pancreas transplantation to help match the donor with the most suitable recipients in order to decrease the likelihood of organ rejection.

[14] 42 U.S.C. § 274(a).

[15] HHS initially published an OPTN final rule on April 2, 1998, 63 Fed. Reg. 16332 (to be codified at 42 C.F.R. pt. 121). The rule was later amended on October 20, 1999 (64 Fed. Reg. 56658), and then became effective on March 16, 2000.

[16] Under a 1986 addition to the Social Security Act, hospitals that participate in Medicare and Medicaid and perform organ transplants are required to be members of and abide by the rules of the OPTN. Pub. L. No. 99-509, § 9318, 100 Stat. 1874, 2009 (adding section 1138 to the Social Security Act) (codified as amended at 42 U.S.C. § 1320b-8). HHS interpreted this provision to require that to be considered a rule or requirement of the OPTN and therefore binding on participating hospitals, the rule or requirement must be formally approved by the Secretary. 54 Fed. Reg. 51802 (Dec. 18, 1989); see also 42 C.F.R. § 121.4(b)(2) and (c) (2007) (regulation providing framework for submission of OPTN policies to the Secretary for review and approval). As of February 2008, the Secretary had not approved any OPTN policies for this purpose. Although OPTN policies have not been formally approved by the Secretary, HRSA has indicated that certain data submitted to the OPTN are mandatory under 42 C.F.R. § 121.11(b)(2) and that failure to submit these data accurately and completely could be considered a violation of this section.

[17] This process is referred to in OPTN policies as confidential medical peer review.

[18] The OPTN contract does not require on-site reviews of kidney transplant programs. Kidney transplant programs are different from other programs in that kidney allocation is determined, in part, by the amount of time the patient

has been waiting, not the severity of the patient's illness. OPTN officials said that kidney transplant programs are reviewed on- site if they are part of a transplant center where the OPTN is reviewing other transplant programs.

[19] Medicare NCDs were published extending coverage to participating and qualified facilities performing heart transplants in 1987, liver transplants in 1991, lung transplants in 1995, pancreas transplants simultaneous with or after kidney transplants in 1999, isolated intestinal and combined liver-intestinal transplants in 2001, and pancreas transplants alone in 2006. 52 Fed. Reg. 10935 (Apr. 6, 1987) (heart); 56 Fed. Reg. 15006 (Apr. 12, 1991) (liver); 60 Fed. Reg. 6537 (Feb. 2, 1995) (lung); CMS Program Memorandum, Transmittal A-99-16 (Apr. 1999) (pancreas simultaneous with or after kidney); CMS Program Memorandum, Transmittal AB-01-58 (Apr. 12, 2001) (intestinal and multivisceral, including combined liver- intestinal); and CMS Pub. 100-03, Transmittal 56 (May 19, 2006) (pancreas). Revised transplant volume requirements for heart, liver, and lung transplant programs were issued on October 11, 2000. CMS Program Memorandum, Transmittal AB-00-95 (Oct. 11, 2000).

[20] See 42 C.F.R. pt. 405, subpt. U (2006).

[21] Most ESRD facilities are renal dialysis facilities, but a small subset of ESRD facilities operate renal transplant programs.

[22] The state agencies are often responsible for surveying other types of health care facilities that require certification for participation in Medicare or Medicaid, such as nursing homes and home health agencies.

[23] CMS initially published a transplant center proposed rule for comment on February 4, 2005. 70 Fed. Reg. 6140. After a comment period, CMS published a final rule on March 30, 2007 (72 Fed. Reg. 15198) (codified at 42. C.F.R. pts. 405, 482, 488, and 498) that became effective on June 28, 2007.

[24] Criteria for Medicare approval differed by program type. In its NCDs, CMS established the criteria that lung and intestine transplant programs should conduct at least 10 transplants per year, and heart and liver transplant programs should conduct at least 12 transplants per year. The criteria for 1-year survival rates for patients after transplantation were 69 percent or higher for lung transplant programs, 65 percent or higher for intestine transplant programs, 73 percent or higher for heart transplant programs, and 77 percent or higher for liver transplant programs.

[25] The earliest possible date of initial Medicare approval was 1986 for heart programs, 1990 for liver programs, 1995 for lung programs, and 2001 for intestine programs.

[26] One CMS regional office reported conducting no complaint investigations of extra-renal transplant programs; another reported that it did not track them. CMS officials also reported conducting several complaint investigations of renal transplant programs.

[27] The Medicare requirements for ESRD facilities addressed issues relevant to all ESRD facilities, such as the maintenance of medical records; they also addressed a limited number of requirements specific to renal transplant programs, such as that the transplant program perform a minimum number of transplants per year, be under the direction of a qualified transplant surgeon or physician, and meet minimal service requirements, including participation in a patient organ allocation registry and provision of social, dietetic, and laboratory services.

[28] See, for example, Institute of Medicine, Organ Procurement and Transplantation: Assessing Current Policies and the Potential Impact of the DHHS Final Rule (Washington, D.C.: National Academies Press, 1999).

[29] Other areas not addressed in the Medicare requirements for ESRD facilities included protections for the safety of living donors, which since 1990 have become the fastest growing source of kidneys for kidney transplants, and implementation of quality assessment and performance improvement programs, now widely used to improve delivery of health care services. CMS recognized the need both to expand and update its requirements for renal and extra-renal transplant programs and to standardize requirements for all types of programs, and began working on new requirements in 2000. CMS had published a proposed version for public comment but had not finalized or implemented these requirements when serious problems came to light in 2005 (the requirements were later finalized in March 2007).

[30] Twenty-seven of the 31 programs were mistakenly classified as no longer participating in Medicare and 4 programs were mistakenly excluded from the survey database. According to CMS officials, the misclassifications likely resulted from state survey agencies mistakenly terminating the ESRD Medicare identification number for the renal transplant program when an associated dialysis program was closed or sold (a renal transplant program and a dialysis program within the same facility were tracked under the same ESRD Medicare identification number). Officials said that this misclassification did not affect renal transplant programs' ability to receive Medicare reimbursement because programs with terminated ESRD identification numbers could continue billing Medicare through their hospital identification numbers.

[31] CMS's goals for ESRD facilities have varied in recent years. For example, in fiscal years 2006 and 2007 CMS had a goal that state agencies assign high priority to surveys of a subset (10 percent) of low-performing ESRD facilities targeted by CMS, as well as a goal that state agencies survey all ESRD facilities every 3.5 years on average; in fiscal years 2004 and 2005 CMS had a goal that state agencies survey all ESRD facilities every 3 years on average.

[32] Until September 2005, the goal to conduct periodic routine on-site reviews was limited to heart and liver programs because patients' priority on the waiting list for these organs depended primarily on medical urgency. The September 2005 OPTN contract incorporated the OPTN's goal of conducting on-site reviews every 3 years and included lung programs in addition to heart and liver programs, after a policy change in which patients' priority on the waiting list for lung transplants would likewise depend upon medical urgency.

[33] The OPTN's monitoring also detected performance problems involving low patient survival rates at another transplant program involved in a high-profile case, although this monitoring did not enable the OPTN to promptly identify the full scope of the problem. (A CMS complaint survey later found that the transplant program did not have a full-time transplant surgeon on staff.)

[34] The period of time ranges from 3 to 12 months, depending on the type of transplant program.

[35] The OPTN had previously identified performance problems at one of these two programs, but the program's survival rates improved and the OPTN released the program from review a few months prior to the time that the staffing problem came to light.

[36] In 2005, the OPTN changed the way it identified programs for additional review. Before 2005, transplant programs flagged as having lower-than-expected outcomes in two consecutive quarterly reports were identified for additional review. As of October 2005, programs flagged as having lower-than-expected outcomes in one report were identified for additional review.

[37] CMS officials reported that they reviewed circumstances at transplant programs on a case-by-case basis to decide which cases constituted egregious noncompliance, and that there were no explicit criteria with which to make this decision.

[38] Transplant programs that were Medicare approved as of June 28, 2007, were required to apply for approval under the new regulations by December 26, 2007, to maintain their Medicare approval until CMS could act on their applications.

[39] According to CMS officials, CMS also plans to monitor compliance with these requirements, and others with which compliance can be monitored using available data, on an ongoing basis during the 3-year approval period.

[40] CMS will consider patient and graft survival rates to be unacceptable if the observed patient or survival rate is lower than expected and all three of the following are true: (1) the one-sided p-value is less than 0.05, (2) the number of observed events (patient deaths or graft failures) minus the number of expected events is greater than 3, and (3) the number of observed events divided by the number of expected events is greater than 1.5.

[41] According to CMS, for initial approval the agency generally will not approve programs that do not meet the data submission, clinical experience, and outcome standards, but the regulations also provide for the consideration of mitigating factors.

[42] Transplant programs that want to continue to be Medicare approved, however, must be in compliance with the new regulations as of June 28, 2007, and must have submitted a request to CMS for Medicare approval under the CoPs no later than December 26, 2007.

[43] On-site surveys in about half of the states will be conducted by state agencies; in the other states, CMS has assigned a contractor to conduct the surveys.

[44] CMS sets priorities for state survey agency workload based on tiers, where Tier 1 is the highest priority and Tier 4 the lowest. In 2007, CMS prioritized surveys of transplant programs at Tier 2.

[45] Another HRSA contractor is providing CMS with quarterly data on transplant programs' survival rates and transplant activity.

[46] 72 Fed. Reg. 15198 (codified in pertinent part at 42 C.F.R. pt. 482, subpt. E).

INDEX

A

B

C

D

H

I

Q

R

S

T